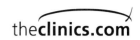

Agnes E. Rupley, DVM, Dipl. ABVP–Avian
CONSULTING EDITOR

VETERINARY CLINICS

OF NORTH AMERICA

Exotic Animal Practice

Toxicology

GUEST EDITOR
Jerry LaBonde, MS, DVM

May 2008 • Volume 11 • Number 2

SAUNDERS

An Imprint of Elsevier, Inc.
PHILADELPHIA   LONDON   TORONTO   MONTREAL   SYDNEY   TOKYO

W.B. SAUNDERS COMPANY
A Division of Elsevier Inc.

Elsevier, Inc., 1600 John F. Kennedy Blvd., Suite 1800, Philadelphia, PA 19103-2899

http://www.vetexotic.theclinics.com

VETERINARY CLINICS OF NORTH AMERICA:	**Volume 11, Number 2**
EXOTIC ANIMAL PRACTICE	**ISSN 1094-9194**
May 2008	**ISBN-13: 978-1-4160-5836-6**
Editor: John Vassallo; j.vassallo@elsevier.com	**ISBN-10: 1-4160-5836-2**

Reprints. For copies of 100 or more of articles in this publication, please contact the commercial Reprints Department, Elsevier Inc., 360 Park Avenue South, New York, New York 10010-1710. Tel: (212) 633-3813 Fax: (212) 633-1935, e-mail: reprints@elsevier.com.

The ideas and opinions expressed in *Veterinary Clinics of North America: Exotic Animal Practice* do not necessarily reflect those of the Publisher. The Publisher does not assume any responsibility for any injury and/or damage to persons or property arising out of or related to any use of the material contained in this periodical. The reader is advised to check the appropriate medical literature and the product information currently provided by the manufacturer of each drug to be administered to verify the dosage, the method and duration of administration, or contraindications. It is the responsibility of the treating physician or other health care professional, relying on independent experience and knowledge of the patient, to determine drug dosages and the best treatment for the patient. Mention of any product in this issue should not be construed as endorsement by the contributors, editors, or the Publisher of the product or manufacturers' claims.

Veterinary Clinics of North America: Exotic Animal Practice (ISSN 1094-9194) is published in January, May, and September by Elsevier, Inc.; Business and Editorial offices: 1600 John F. Kennedy Blvd., Suite 1800, Philadelphia, PA 19103-2899. Customer Service Office: 6277 Sea Harbor Drive, Orlando, FL 32887-4800. Subscription prices are $161.00 per year for US individuals, $288.00 per year for US institutions, $84.00 per year for US students and residents, $190.00 per year for Canadian individuals, $333.00 per year for Canadian institutions, $202.00 per year for international individuals, $333.00 per year for international institutions and $101.00 per year for Canadian and foreign students/residents. To receive student/resident rate, orders must be accompanied by name of affiliated institution, date of term, and the *signature* of program/residency coordinator on institution letterhead. Orders will be billed at individual rate until proof of status is received. Foreign air speed delivery is included in all *Clinics* subscription prices. All prices are subject to change without notice.

POSTMASTER: Send address changes to *Veterinary Clinics of North America: Exotic Animal Practice*; Elsevier Periodicals Customer Service, 6277 Sea Harbor Drive, Orlando, FL 32887-4800. **Customer Service: 1-800-654-2452 (US). From outside of the United States, call 1-407-563-6020. Fax: 1-407-363-9661. E-mail: JournalsCustomerService-usa@elsevier.com.**

Veterinary Clinics of North America: Exotic Animal Practice is covered in *Index Medicus*.

Printed in the United States of America.

CONSULTING EDITOR

AGNES E. RUPLEY, DVM, Diplomate, American Board of Veterinary Practitioners–Avian; Director and Chief Veterinarian, All Pets Medical & Laser Surgical Center, College Station, Texas

GUEST EDITOR

JERRY LABONDE, MS, DVM, Avian and Exotic Animal Hospital at Homestead, Centennial, Colorado

CONTRIBUTORS

LORI R. ARENT, BS, MS, Clinic Manager, The Raptor Center, College of Veterinary Medicine, University of Minnesota, St. Paul, Minnesota

KEITH BOESEN, PharmD, Arizona Poison and Drug Information Center, College of Pharmacy, University of Arizona, Tucson, Arizona

LESLIE BOYER, MD, Fellow, American College of Medical Toxicology; Arizona Poison and Drug Information Center, College of Pharmacy, University of Arizona, Tucson, Arizona

LAUREL A. DEGERNES, DVM, MPH, Diplomate, American Board of Veterinary Practitioners–Avian; Associate Professor of Avian Medicine and Epidemiology, Department of Clinical Sciences, College of Veterinary Medicine, North Carolina State University, Raleigh, North Carolina

ERIC DUNAYER, MS, VMD, Diplomate, American Board of Toxicology; Diplomate, American Board of Veterinary Toxicology; Senior Toxicologist, American Society for the Prevention of Cruelty to Animals (ASPCA) Animal Poison Control Center (APCC); Adjunct Instructor, College of Veterinary Medicine, University of Illinois, Urbana, Illinois

KEVIN T. FITZGERALD, PhD, DVM, Diplomate, American Board of Veterinary Practitioners; Staff Veterinarian, Alameda East Veterinary Hospital, Denver, Colorado

MATTHEW S. JOHNSTON, VMD, Diplomate, American Board of Veterinary Practitioners–Avian; Assistant Professor of Zoological Medicine, James L. Voss Veterinary Teaching Hospital, Colorado State University, Fort Collins, Colorado

MARLA LICHTENBERGER, DVM, Diplomate, American College of Veterinary Emergency and Critical Care; Milwaukee Emergency Clinic for Animals and Specialty Services, Milwaukee, Wisconsin

TERESA L. LIGHTFOOT, DVM, Diplomate, American Board of Veterinary Practitioners–Avian; Department of Avian and Exotic Medicine, Florida Veterinary Specialists, Tampa, Florida

JUDE MCNALLY, RPh, Diplomate, American Board of Applied Toxicology; Arizona Poison and Drug Information Center, College of Pharmacy, University of Arizona, Tucson, Arizona

KRISTIN L. NEWQUIST, BS, AAS, CVT, Exotic Animal Technician, Alameda East Veterinary Hospital, Denver, Colorado

BRIAN S. PALMEIRO, VMD, PetFishDoctor.com, Prospect Park, Pennsylvania

MICHAEL E. PETERSON, DVM, MS, Staff Veterinarian, Reid Veterinary Hospital, Albany; Instructor, College of Veterinary Medicine, Oregon State University, Corvallis, Oregon

ROBERT H. POPPENGA, DVM, PhD, Diplomate, American Board of Veterinary Toxicology; California Animal Health and Food Safety Laboratory, School of Veterinary Medicine, University of California, Davis, California

PATRICK T. REDIG, DVM, PhD, Professor, The Raptor Center, College of Veterinary Medicine, University of Minnesota, St. Paul, Minnesota

JILL A. RICHARDSON, DVM, The Hartz Mountain Corporation; Consultant, Toxicology Boards, Veterinary Information Network, Secaucus, New Jersey

HELEN ROBERTS, DVM, Aquatic Veterinary Services of WNY, 5 Corners Animal Hospital, Orchard Park, New York

JULIE M. YEAGER, DVM, Department of Avian and Exotic Medicine, Florida Veterinary Specialists, Tampa, Florida

CONTENTS

> A toxicologic diagnosis is based on knowledge of the circum-
> stances surrounding a particular case, knowledge of the clinical
> symptomatology, receipt and evaluation of proper specimens by a
> qualified laboratory, and judicious interpretation of the laboratory
> results. Failure to have all necessary ingredients can result in a
> wrong or missed diagnosis. Many veterinary toxicology laborato-
> ries can detect suspected toxicants in feed, tissue, and environ-
> mental samples at extremely low concentrations. The ability to
> detect toxicants at such low levels has often outpaced the ability of
> the diagnostician to interpret the analytic findings. This article
> provides guidelines for acquiring a good history, collecting
> appropriate samples for analysis, and selecting a veterinary
> analytic laboratory to maximize the probability of making a correct
> toxicologic diagnosis.

> The poisoned exotic veterinary patient remains a significant
> challenge to the clinician. A patient presenting with the history
> of exposure to a toxin or poison should be considered to have a
> potentially life-threatening problem. This article details the ABCs
> of emergency medicine including fluid therapy and discusses the
> principles of neurologic management. The last part of the article
> provides the clinician with guidelines for decontamination and
> critical care management of some of the more common toxicoses in
> exotic animals.

information on specific toxicants in ferrets. This article initially reviews general consideration in treating poisoning in ferrets, such as obtaining history and decontamination. It then discusses some specific agents that appear to be common causes of poisoning in ferrets based on the experience of the ASPCA Animal Poison Control Center.

Toxicoses are an uncommon presentation to rabbit practitioners; however, veterinarians who accept rabbits as patients should be familiar with the basic concepts of toxicosis management and the specific syndromes associated with clinical toxicoses. The objective of this article is to present clinically relevant information for veterinarians presented with rabbits exhibiting characteristic signs of toxicosis. In addition, specific mention is made to the most common clinical toxicoses, including lead, chemicals, rodenticides, aflatoxins, and poisonous plants.

Reptiles are increasingly being kept as pets in American households. The basic principles of emergency medicine are the same for all species, but reptilian species present special diagnostic challenges to veterinary clinicians when they become ill. Reptiles in captivity can become accidentally poisoned in a variety of ways. Veterinarians treating small animal emergencies must make an effort to familiarize themselves with the large body of literature and resources that are developing regarding both nontraditional exotic companion species and advances in toxicology.

Most aquarium fish live in a closed system, so the effects of toxins can be cumulative and devastating. Most cases of toxicity are due to deficiencies in husbandry and tank maintenance. Poor water quality kills more fish than infectious agents, making client education a very important preventive tool for aquatic practitioners. This article includes a discussion of toxicities related to water quality, chemotherapeutics, pesticides, and household substances.

The purpose of this article is to familiarize the reader with the basic venom components, the pathophysiologic responses of

envenomated dogs and cats, and some brief treatment guidelines
for envenomations by various exotic "pets." Representative toxic
species of reptiles, amphibians, and arthropods are included. The
growing trend toward the collection of exotic animals by private
owners increases the likelihood that veterinarians will face the
challenge of treating an exotic envenomation.

Toxicologic Information Resources for Reptile Envenomations 389
Jude McNally, Keith Boesen, and Leslie Boyer

The United States is the largest importer of reptiles in the world,
with an estimated 1.5 to 2.0 million households keeping one or
more reptiles. Snakes account for about 11% of these imports and it
has been estimated that as many as 9% of these reptiles are
venomous. Envenomations by nonindigenous venomous species
are a rare but often serious medical emergency. Bites may occur
during the care and handling of legitimate collections found in
universities, zoos, or museums. The other predominant source of
exotic envenomation is from amateur collectors participating in
importation, propagation, and trade of non-native species. This
article provides toxicologic information resources for snake
envenomations.

FORTHCOMING ISSUES

RECENT ISSUES

The Clinics are now available online!

Access your subscription at
www.theclinics.com

VETERINARY
CLINICS
Exotic Animal Practice

Vet Clin Exot Anim 11 (2008) xi–xii

Preface

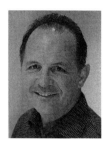

Jerry LaBonde, MS, DVM
Guest Editor

The passion of veterinary medicine is the lifelong commitment to improve our level of knowledge so we can provide a greater service to our patients and their human guardians. This commitment has always been a difficult task for the exotic animal veterinarian. The large number of different species we see and the limited number of resources (especially in toxicology) have made this problematic in the past. The availability of quality exotic animal veterinary resources is much better today; however, there has never been a single toxicology text that addressed most of the exotic animal species seen by the exotic animal veterinarian. In this issue of *Veterinary Clinics of North America: Exotic Animal Practice*, we have filled that void and provided a single go-to reference on toxicology of exotic animals.

The authors were chosen for their professionalism, expertise, and clinical experience. Their articles went beyond my expectations, providing a solid foundation of toxicologic information with many unique and insightful perspectives on their topics. This issue begins with the all important basics of diagnostic sampling and establishing a minimum database, followed by critical care of the toxicology patient. The articles following address the different exotic animals and their toxicologic conditions. There are an endless number of potential toxicants that exotic animals could be exposed to. The authors have compiled the most common and relevant information related to the toxicology for their species.

The exotic animal veterinarian is also faced with the handling and treatment of venomous species in which we, our patients, or their owners may be exposed to these animals' toxins. For that reason, articles on "Toxic

doi:10.1016/j.cvex.2008.01.007

Exotics" and "Toxicologic Information Resources for Reptile Envenomations" have been included.

I would like to thank all of the authors for their commitment and wisdom
in putting together this unique source of information for the exotic animal
veterinarian. I would also like to thank Elsevier and *Veterinary Clinics of
North America: Exotic Animal Practice* for their dedication and support
of the exotic animal veterinarian.

Jerry LaBonde, MS, DVM
Avian and Exotic Animal Hospital at Homestead
6900 South Holly Circle
Centennial, CO 80112, USA

E-mail address: labonde14@aol.com

ELSEVIER
SAUNDERS

VETERINARY
CLINICS
Exotic Animal Practice

Vet Clin Exot Anim 11 (2008) 195–210

Diagnostic Sampling and Establishing a Minimum Database in Exotic Animal Toxicology

Robert H. Poppenga, DVM, PhD, DABVT

*California Animal Health and Food Safety Laboratory, School of Veterinary Medicine,
University of California, West Health Sciences Drive, Davis, CA 95616, USA*

The establishment of a toxicologic diagnosis requires the same approach as that for any nontoxicologic diagnosis: obtaining a comprehensive history, establishing a minimum database, collection of appropriate samples for analysis, and correct interpretation of laboratory results. In suspected intoxications, three scenarios are possible: an asymptomatic or symptomatic animal has been exposed to a known toxicant, an asymptomatic or symptomatic animal has been exposed to an unidentified toxicant, or an animal is showing clinical signs due to an unknown cause for which toxicants should be included in a differential diagnosis [1]. In many situations, a client calls asking whether an asymptomatic animal should be examined following a known ingestion of a chemical. In such situations, establishment of an exposure dose, if possible, and comparison of the exposure dose with specific toxicity information about a chemical is a critical first step in deciding subsequent advice (eg, observing the animal at home or bringing the animal to the hospital for possible decontamination).

Case history

A proper history is an essential first ingredient for a successful toxicologic diagnosis. A good clinical history may provide specific clues or may only point the veterinarian and the diagnostician in a general direction. A good clinical history includes animal signalment, a thorough description of clinical signs, if observed, husbandry practices, environmental conditions, and possible chemical exposures. Notation of preexisting health problems is also important since underlying disease processes can contribute to increased sensitivity of an animal to a chemical. Important historical

---

E-mail address: rhpoppenga@ucdavis.edu

doi:10.1016/j.cvex.2008.01.005

information includes the following: breed; sex; age; weight; current medical treatments, including any dietary supplements or herbs; number of animals in the group; number of animals affected; number potentially exposed; number exhibiting clinical signs; type, duration, and severity of signs; possible time of exposure to identified chemicals; degree of exposure (dose) if known or if worst case estimates can be made; and chemical formulations if possible [1–4]. If an animal has been exposed or potentially exposed to an identified product, and a decision is made that the exposure is clinically significant, it is always recommended that the product be brought to the clinic for inspection if it can be handled in a safe manner. Examination of product labels can assist in the exposure assessment and provide a phone number if additional information about the product is needed.

It is important that the veterinarian not be misled by the perceptions of the owner. In many cases, owners are convinced that their animal has been "poisoned." This statement can lead many veterinarians to consider only a toxicologic etiology in lieu of other infectious or noninfectious causes of illness. Alternatively, the veterinarian should be careful in suggesting to a client that his or her animal appears to have been poisoned, when inadequate evidence exists to support such a conclusion.

Suspected cases of intoxication are often emotional and potentially involve litigation, especially when affected animals are rare and/or valuable. Because of the potential for litigation, it is incumbent upon the veterinarian to document all procedures and consider following a chain-of-custody process for all samples. Proper chain-of-custody involves creating a paper trail for each sample that documents in detail how a sample was stored, shipped, tested, and discarded.

Clinical signs

Clinical signs may lead the veterinarian to suspect a particular toxicant. For example, the cholinesterase-inhibiting organophosphorus (OP) and carbamate insecticides often cause characteristic clinical signs that can be remembered by the mnemonic DUMBELS for diarrhea, urination, miosis, bronchospasm, emesis, lacrimation, and salivation, respectively. Alternatively, clinical signs may be rather nonspecific and therefore of less help. Clinical pathologic results can provide important clues to possible toxicant exposure and can influence the decontamination procedure employed, early use of antidotes, list of differential diagnoses, and choice of analytic tests. For example, the presence of metabolic acidosis and high anion and osmolal gaps suggest ethylene glycol or methanol toxicoses. The presence of prolonged clotting times are compatible with exposure to an anticoagulant rodenticide. Unfortunately, most toxicants do not result in characteristic clinical pathologic changes; however, the identification of affected organs can often narrow a list of differentials since many toxicants affect only one or two organ systems.

Establishing a minimum database

Routine laboratory testing is recommended for all suspected life-threatening intoxications [5]. The components of a minimum toxicologic database include complete blood count (CBC); serum electrolytes; arterial blood gas analysis; pulse oximetry; serum glucose; BUN (blood urea nitrogen); creatinine, calcium, and liver enzyme determinations; and a urinalysis. Depending on the clinical signs exhibited and physical examination findings, tests such as a coagulation panel or electrocardiography can be warranted. Radiographs should be considered as part of the minimum database (especially in birds or exotic animals kept in enclosures accessible by the public) to rule out the presence of metallic objects in the gastrointestinal (GI) tract.

Postmortem examination

In many toxicoses, the only clinical sign is death. A thorough postmortem examination is essential in such circumstances. This may help eliminate nontoxicologic etiologies or perhaps narrow the list of possible toxicants. It should be kept in mind that many toxic agents may cause nonspecific lesions or no lesions at all.

Often, when a postmortem examination is done in the clinic, tissue samples are collected for either histologic or toxicologic examination, but not both. Two sets of tissue samples from animals with suspected toxicoses should be routinely saved. One set should be preserved in 10% buffered formalin for histologic evaluation and another set frozen for possible toxicologic analysis. A common and often unforgiving mistake is failure to submit brain, spinal cord, or peripheral nervous tissue when signs referable to the central or peripheral nervous system are present. A prudent and cost-effective procedure in unexplained deaths is to submit a full set of tissues for histologic examination following gross examination and to keep a second set frozen for later toxicologic analysis pending the histologic findings. It is always easier to dispose of unneeded frozen tissues than to collect tissues from an animal that has already been buried or otherwise discarded.

Ideally, a complete postmortem examination should be conducted by a board-certified pathologist at an accredited veterinary diagnostic laboratory with toxicologic testing capabilities. A list of accredited veterinary diagnostic laboratories can be found on the American Association of Veterinary Laboratory Diagnostician's Web site at http://www.aavld.org/mc/page.do. Links to individual laboratories are provided. Some laboratories accept only certain animal species for evaluation and not all laboratories have toxicologic testing capabilities. Therefore, it is always useful to call the laboratory for specific information relating to the case at hand.

Sample collection and submission

General sample collection protocols for investigation of possible toxicoses when live and/or dead animals are involved have been published [2–4]. Additional comments on selected samples can be found in Table 1. Noteworthy are the references to urine and crop contents, which are samples that are often overlooked, but may sometimes be the most important to obtaining a diagnosis. Also, if an animal has vomited in the home environment, it can be critical that the owner bring a sample with the animal if a judgment is made that an animal should be examined.

It is critical that samples are stored and shipped appropriately. Specimens should not be submitted in containers that have been used previously to store other materials, even if believed to be clean. When multiple samples are submitted, each container should be labeled with the name of the animal, the name of the owner, the date of collection, and the identification of the specimen.

Depending on the toxicant of interest, samples should be either refrigerated or frozen. Refrigeration is generally sufficient if samples are to be shipped and tested soon after collection. If samples are to be retained pending other testing, freezing is more appropriate. When shipping samples, leak-proof packaging and appropriate cooling are required. With a few possible exceptions, using ice packs provides sufficient cooling. Samples should be packaged in a way that avoids cross-contamination. Concentrated chemical sources such as bait formulations or other products (ie, sprays, liquids, powders) can potentially leak through plastic bags; in such cases wrapping the sample in aluminum foil or placing in a separate metal container may be warranted. Use overnight delivery services, but avoid shipping samples to arrive on weekends or holidays, since the package can sit for a period of time before processing. Follow all applicable regulations regarding shipment of biological samples.

Toxicology laboratory testing

It is advisable to be familiar with the testing procedures of the diagnostic laboratory that you use. Although most laboratories offer a wide range of analytic tests, no one laboratory can run all possible analyses. If a particular test is not offered by an individual laboratory, it may be possible to forward the sample to a referral laboratory. Laboratory personnel are often knowledgeable about which laboratories have the capability and expertise to run an unusual test. The frequency of particular toxicoses varies for different regions of the country and thus the need for investing the resources and manpower to develop specific testing capabilities also varies. Generally, it is not cost-effective for diagnostic laboratories to develop analytic procedures for which they receive few requests, although some laboratories are willing to develop new chemical assays depending on their resources and circumstances of the case. Thus, lists of tests provided on Web sites or in users' guides may not always reflect what a laboratory is willing to or capable of providing.

Since many analytic procedures can detect the presence of certain compounds over a wide range of tissue concentrations, toxicology laboratories are not necessarily restricted to detection of high, potentially toxic concentrations of these agents. For example, some toxicology laboratories may offer therapeutic drug monitoring services or determinations of tissue mineral concentrations to rule out deficiency diseases.

The sophistication of analytic systems has enabled the diagnostic toxicologist to look for literally thousands of chemical compounds with a high degree of specificity and sensitivity. In cases in which there is no history of exposure to specific chemicals, powerful screening tools such as gas chromatography–mass spectrometry (GC/MS) and inductively coupled argon plasma emission spectroscopy (ICPAES) are available to detect a broad array of inorganic and organic compounds, respectively. For example, some diagnostic laboratories, using ICPAES or another metal-screening technique called inductively coupled plasma mass spectrometry (ICP/MS), can test for several dozen metals with one analysis in tissue, fluid, and environmental samples.

Sample size or type can be the limiting factors in the ability of a laboratory to test for a large number of compounds. Small sample sizes limit the number of tests that can be performed and can also decrease the sensitivity of a particular analytic technique. For example, if an analytic procedure typically requires 1 g of tissue to maximize sensitivity, the availability of only 0.5 gram can decrease the sensitivity of the test by a factor of two.

It is important to note that, for certain toxicants, it is not necessary to quantify tissue concentrations; the presence of detectable toxicant in tissues along with compatible clinical signs is sufficient to yield a diagnosis. Alternatively, for agents that are ubiquitous in the environment, quantification of tissue concentrations may be critical for proper differentiation of a toxicosis from a background exposure.

Specific toxicants (Table 2)

Metals

Lead

Analysis of lead is one of the more commonly requested diagnostic tests. Fortunately, lead analysis can be done on small sample sizes and is widely available. Antemortem, whole blood is the sample of choice since lead associates almost exclusively with the red blood cell. Neither serum nor plasma are appropriate samples for testing. The type of anticoagulant used to preserve whole blood does not affect laboratory results in most cases, but it is always recommended to call the laboratory when in doubt. Liver or kidney samples are the preferred postmortem samples.

Table 1
Comments on selected specimens for submission to veterinary toxicology laboratories

Specimen	Ideal sample amount[a]	Comments and special considerations
Urine[b]	10 mL; store in nonbreakable, leak-proof container.	Underutilized sample The pharmacokinetics of a particular compound need to be considered to assess its utility Possible to identify chemicals in urine that cannot be detected in other tissue or fluid samples Best used to indicate exposure; more difficult to interpret the significance of quantitative results Recommended quantity can be difficult to obtain from small animals
Kidney	2 to 10 g Store and submit frozen unless testing soon after collection in which case refrigeration is appropriate	Best tissue to submit in certain heavy metal intoxications (lead, arsenic, mercury) Tissue of choice for calcium determinations in suspected ethylene glycol exposures Can be used for organic chemical screening, but liver is preferred
Liver	2 to 10 g Store and submit frozen unless testing soon after collection in which case refrigeration is appropriate	Perhaps the best tissue specimen for general mineral or organic chemical screening tests
Vomitus, stomach/crop and intestinal contents	2 to 10 g Store and submit frozen unless testing soon after collection in which case refrigeration is appropriate	Can find the highest concentrations of rapidly acting toxicants in stomach or crop samples Owner should be instructed to save vomitus if animal has vomited before presentation If gastric lavage is performed in hospital, save initial lavage material for testing Can be combined or pooled from several affected animals if sample quantities are limiting
Tissue surrounding suspected injection site	1 g Store and submit frozen unless testing soon after collection in which case refrigeration is appropriate	Can provide a specimen containing a high concentration of a chemical

Sample	Recommendations	Comments
Brain	For larger animals, make a midsagittal cut to submit half of brain; for small animals and most birds, submit entire brain, especially if not needed for other diagnostic purposes. Store and submit frozen unless testing soon after collection	Used primarily for determination of cholinesterase activity. Cholinesterase activities vary among different brain regions; most laboratories use one entire half to ensure consistency of results. Can also be used to diagnose intoxication due to organochlorine insecticides or macrolide endectocides
Fat	2 to 10 g	Useful for detection of some fat-soluble chemicals such as OCs, PCBs, and bromethalin
Bedding	100-g representative sample	Submit sample from cage and a separate sample from the original container if possible
Water	1 L in a clean, leakproof container	Large volumes are generally needed due to relatively low concentrations of toxicants that can be present. One of the most important samples for investigating fish problems
Samples of medications, commercial products or baits	Store and submit frozen unless testing soon after collection in which case refrigeration is appropriate. No firm rule for amount to submit; generally 2 to 3 tablets or capsules of a medication; 50 to 100 g of a solid material or bait; 20 to 100 mL of a liquid (mix liquid before sampling to ensure a representative sample)	Relatively small sample sizes are needed due to high concentrations of chemicals present. Analysis can help confirm the identity of an unknown chemical present in a sample
Cage material or toys	Several small pieces are generally sufficient for metal testing	Primarily used to confirm the presence of metals such as lead and zinc

Abbreviation: OC, organochlorine.

[a] In general, always strive to submit as much sample as possible. Sample sizes smaller than those recommended can be diagnostic; it is always good to consult with the laboratory to discuss potential limitations of less than recommended sample sizes. In some cases, small samples from more than one affected individual can be pooled for analysis.

[b] While not commonly submitted, bird droppings may be useful.

Table 2
Appropriate sampling for specific toxicants

Test	Preferred specimens and minimum specimen amounts	Storing and shipping container	Additional comments
Amanitin (toxin found in *Amanita* spp. mushrooms)	10 g GI contents	Whirlpac bag or screw-cap container for GI contents or urine	The test is qualitative in nature meaning that it is reported as either positive or negative
	2 mL urine 1 mL serum Mushroom	Vacutainer or plastic tube for serum Paper bag for mushroom	Experts generally need to be consulted for positive mushroom identification
Anticoagulant rodenticides	10 g liver	Whirlpac bag or screw-cap container for tissues or bait	Several anticoagulant rodenticides are typically included in analytic screens. Results can be qualitative or quantitative.
	1 mL whole blood or serum 10 g of bait	Vacutainer or plastic tube for whole blood or serum	
Arsenic	10 g liver or kidney	Whirlpac bag or screw-cap container for tissues, urine, GI contents, or source material	Kidney cortex is preferred specimen; arsenic is eliminated quickly, so if there is a delay between exposure and sample collection, urine is likely to be the best sample.
	1 mL whole blood 2 mL urine 5 g GI contents Source material	Vacutainer or plastic tube for whole blood	
Avicides (Starlicide or Avitrol)	5 g GI contents Source material	Whirlpac bag or screw-cap container for GI contents or source material	
Bromethalin	5 g fat, brain, or liver	Whirlpac bag or screw-cap container for tissues or source material	
Carbamate insecticides	10 g GI contents, liver, or source material	Whirlpac bag or screw-cap container for GI contents, tissues, or source material	Make sure that sample cross-contamination does not occur; use of aluminum foil or metal containers should be considered
	1 mL blood or serum	Vacutainer tube or plastic capped vial for blood or serum	Whole blood or brain should be submitted as well for cholinesterase activity determination

Toxin	Sample required	Container	Comments
Cyanide	2 g of muscle, liver, or GI contents	Whirlpac bag or screw-cap container for GI contents, tissues, or source material	Samples should be frozen in an airtight container as soon as possible and shipped to arrive frozen at the laboratory due to the volatility of cyanide
	2 mL of whole blood; 10 g of feed or plant material; 10 mL water	Vacutainer tube for blood or serum	
Drugs (OTC, prescription, or illicit)	10 g liver	Whirlpac bag or screw-cap container for tissue	Calling laboratory before submission is recommended to ensure that analytic test is available if there is a specific drug of concern
	As much urine as is available	Leakproof container for urine	
	2 mL of serum or plasma	Vacutainer tube or plastic capped vial for serum or plasma	
Ethylene glycol	10 g liver or kidney	Whirlpac bag or screw-cap container for tissues or source material	
	1 mL serum or plasma; 1 g of source material	Vacutainer tube for serum or plasma	
Lead	1 mL whole blood	Whirlpac bag or screw-cap container for tissues; vacutainer tube for whole blood	In general, the anticoagulant used (heparin, EDTA, etc.) does not affect the analysis. When in doubt, call the laboratory before blood collection.
	1 g liver or kidney		If sending kidney, cortex is preferred
	1 mL whole blood		If sending kidney, cortex is preferred
Mercury	1 g liver or kidney	Whirlpac bag or screw-cap container for tissues	
	1 mL urine	Leakproof container for urine	
		Vacutainer tube for whole blood	
Metaldehyde	1 g stomach contents or source material	Whirlpac bag or screw-cap container for stomach contents or source material	
	2 mL urine; 1 mL serum or plasma	Leakproof container for urine; vacutainer tube for serum or plasma	

(continued on next page)

Table 2 (*continued*)

Test	Preferred specimens and minimum specimen amounts	Storing and shipping container	Additional comments
Metal screens	1 g of liver or kidney	Whirlpac bag or screw-cap container for tissues, source materials, or objects	Keep in mind that rubber can leach zinc and possibly contaminate sample if it comes into contact with the rubber; particularly of concern with serum or plasma samples
	5 g source material, feed, or metallic object	Leakproof container for urine and water	
	2 mL whole blood or serum/plasma	Vacutainer tube for serum, plasma, or whole blood	
	2 to 10 mL urine		
	50 mL of water		
Microcystins	5 g GI contents	Whirlpac bag or screw-cap container for GI contents or bloom material	A sample of bloom material should be placed in 10% formalin for identification of algae as well
	Minimum of 5 mL of water	Leakproof container for water	
	5 g algal blood material		
Mycotoxins	50 g of feed	If feed sample is dry, it can be placed in a paper bag and kept at ambient temperature	Biologic samples are generally not very useful for diagnosing mycotoxin problems. The one exception is for the tremorgenic toxin, penitrem A: source material (ie, moldy dairy product or compost sample) and GI contents (1 g), serum (1 mL), and urine (1 mL) can be submitted.
		If feed sample is moist, can be placed in a plastic bag and kept frozen	
Oleandrin (*Nerium oleander*)	5 g GI contents, liver, or plant material	Whirlpac bag or screw-cap container for GI contents or tissues	
	1 mL serum or plasma	Vacutainer tube for serum or plasma	
		No special container for plant material	
Organochlorine insecticides	1 g liver, fat, or brain	Whirlpac bag or screw-cap container for tissues or source material	Make sure that sample cross-contamination does not occur; use of aluminum foil or metal containers should be considered
	1 g source material	Vacutainer tube for whole blood	
	1 mL whole blood		

Organophosphorus insecticides	10 g GI contents, liver, or source material	Whirlpac bag or screw-cap container for GI contents, tissues, or source material	Make sure that sample cross-contamination does not occur; use of aluminum foil or metal containers should be considered
	1 mL blood or serum	Vacutainer tube or plastic capped vial for blood or serum	Whole blood or brain should be submitted as well for cholinesterase activity determination
Paraquat	5 g lung, GI contents, or source material	Whirlpac bag or screw-cap container for GI contents, tissues, or source material	Residues of the parent compound appear to be the most persistent in lung tissue, which is the principal target organ for paraquat toxicity
	2 mL urine	Leakproof container for urine	
	2 mL serum or plasma	Vacutainer tube or plastic capped vial for serum or plasma	
Polychlorinated hydrocarbons (PCBs)	1 g liver, fat, or brain	Whirlpac bag or screw-cap container for tissues or source material	Make sure that sample cross-contamination does not occur; use of aluminum foil or metal containers should be considered
	1 g source material		
	1 mL whole blood	Vacutainer tube for whole blood	
Plant ID	Entire plant or as much of a plant as possible	Plant can be dried or fresh; if fresh, the roots of the plant should be wrapped in a wet paper towel, placed in a plastic bag, and kept refrigerated	Do not freeze the plant: submission of only plant fragments makes identification more difficult, although plant fragments collected from the stomach should be submitted for possible gross or microscopic identification
Pyrethrin or pyrethroid insecticides	5 g of GI contents, liver, source material, or feed	Whirlpac bag or screw-cap container for GI contents, tissues, source material, or feed	Make sure that sample cross-contamination does not occur; use of aluminum foil or metal containers should be considered
	1 mL of serum	Vacutainer tube or plastic capped vial for serum or plasma	
Selenium	1 g of liver or kidney	Whirlpac bag or screw-cap container for tissues or feed	
	10 g of feed	Leakproof container for urine or water	

(continued on next page)

Table 2 (*continued*)

Test	Preferred specimens and minimum specimen amounts	Storing and shipping container	Additional comments
	1 mL whole blood or serum/plasma	Vacutainer tube for whole blood, serum, or plasma	
	5 mL urine		
	10 mL water		
Strychnine	1 g GI contents, liver, or source material	Whirlpac bag or screw-cap container for tissues, GI contents, or source material	
	1 mL serum/plasma	Leakproof container for urine	
	1 mL urine	Vacutainer tube for serum or plasma	
Thallium	1 g liver or kidney	Whirlpac bag or screw-cap container for tissues	
	1 mL whole blood or urine	Leakproof container for urine	
		Vacutainer tube for whole blood	
Vitamin A	1 g liver	Whirlpac bag or screw-cap container for tissues or feed	Minimize contact with light (serum/plasma tubes should be wrapped in aluminum foil). Keep well chilled or frozen at all times.
	1 mL serum or plasma	Vacutainer tube for serum or plasma	
	3 g feed		
Zinc or aluminum phosphide	1 g GI contents, source material, or feed	Whirlpac bag or screw-cap container for GI contents, source material, or feed	Samples should be kept tightly sealed and well chilled since phosphene, generated from zinc or aluminum phosphide, is volatile

Abbreviations: GI, gastrointestinal; OTC, over-the-counter.

Zinc

Zinc determination is another commonly requested test. In contrast to lead, serum or plasma are the specimens of choice for analysis. There are two notes of caution concerning zinc. First, rubber can leach significant amounts of zinc [6]. Therefore, royal blue Vacutainer tubes or plastic vials with plastic caps are recommended for sample collection and storage. Sample hemolysis can also result in artificial increases in serum or plasma zinc concentrations. Second, there is evidence that serum or plasma zinc concentrations show diurnal variation [7]. Thus, interpretation of single, moderately elevated zinc concentrations as evidence for exposure to excessive zinc needs to be done cautiously.

Occasionally, diagnostic laboratories are asked to test hair for the diagnosis of metal intoxications or deficiencies. Except for infrequent instances of documenting exposure to certain metals such as lead, mercury, arsenic, or thallium or some organic compounds, routine use of hair for toxicologic analyses is not routinely useful.

Insecticides

Cholinesterase-inhibiting insecticides

This group includes the OP and carbamate insecticides. Stomach or crop contents and (less often) liver and skin or hair are the samples most likely to yield positive results when submitted in an attempt to determine the presence of a specific compound. Some OPs and most carbamates are rapidly metabolized and eliminated from tissues, and it is not unusual to fail to detect them except in cases of acute death following exposure. Cholinesterase determinations on whole-blood or brain samples are often valuable adjunctive tests in cases of suspected OP toxicosis, owing to the relatively tight and persistent binding of the enzyme and resultant inhibition of its activity by these compounds. Carbamates only transiently bind cholinesterase and therefore depression of enzyme activity is not as consistent as in the case of OP toxicoses. Following exposure to carbamates, it is possible to have initially inhibited enzyme activity that returns to normal during shipment of a sample to the laboratory.

It is important to recognize that different methodologies for measuring cholinesterase activity generally make interlaboratory comparisons of cholinesterase values inappropriate. In addition, there are marked species differences with regard to normal cholinesterase activities in a given tissue, and the sensitivity among species of the cholinesterase enzymes in red blood cells and plasma to inhibition by OPs or carbamates varies. Acetylcholinesterase activity also varies in different regions of the brain. Generally, one half of the brain, divided midsagittally, is submitted to the laboratory for analysis to minimize sample variation. Some laboratories require the caudate nucleus and base their interpretations on only this portion of the brain. Because of these considerations, it is important for the laboratory performing the analyses to have a database of normal versus depressed levels for a range of species, and, generally, these must be determined in each laboratory, using the method they routinely employ. Cholinesterase activity should not be the only criterion used for evaluating a case of suspected OP or carbamate toxicosis. It is best to check with your laboratory when submitting any specimen for the first time.

Pyrethrin and pyrethroid insecticides

This group of insecticides is widely used for a variety of purposes. Many of these insecticides can be detected in tissues such as the brain and liver. Unfortunately, interpretation of detected tissue concentrations is still very difficult in assessing suspected toxicoses. Until more information is available relating tissue concentrations to adverse effects, analytic tests will be valuable only for confirming exposures and for serving as a developing database of values associated with clinical signs or death.

On occasion, synergists such as piperonyl butoxide or MGK 264 are detected in tissue samples. Since these compounds are frequently a component of insecticidal formulations containing pyrethrins or pyrethroids and less frequently a component of other insecticide formulations, their presence can be a clue to previous exposure to this insecticide category.

Organochlorine insectides

Although not as commonly encountered today as several years ago, occasional acute exposures of wildlife to organochlorine (OC; chlorinated hydrocarbon) insecticides still occur. These compounds are extremely lipid-soluble and tend to concentrate in highest amounts in adipose tissue. Other organs such as the brain and liver can accumulate OCs, but concentrations tend to be much lower than in adipose tissue. The OC insecticides are still commonly detected, often at nontoxic concentrations in certain wild animals, particularly birds. From a live animal, the specimens of choice for OC analysis are body fat and serum. Brain, liver, and body fat can be submitted from dead animals. Because of the possibility of redistribution to fat that may occur to a limited extent in acute exposures or to a very great degree in chronic exposures, brain concentrations of the OC compounds, which correlate with the occurrence of neurologic signs, are of greatest importance in diagnosis. Body fat and liver concentrations are often much more difficult to interpret. It is important to note whether results are reported on a tissue wet weight basis or tissue fat basis, since the numerical values from the same tissue are considerably different.

Rodenticides

Anticoagulant rodenticides remain a common toxicologic problem in some animal species. Of particular concern for wildlife and exotic species that feed on small rodents is the possibility of secondary intoxication from anticoagulant rodenticide residues in food items. It is critical that exotic pet owners know the source of the food items that they provide to their animals to ensure that they are chemical free. When intoxication is suspected in a live animal, whole blood or serum can be submitted for analysis. If the animal dies, analysis of liver tissue or unclotted blood is generally recommended. Stomach contents are often submitted in lieu of other tissues, but they are often not the best choice given the delay of 48 to 72 hours between possible exposure and the onset of clinical signs.

Natural toxins

There are a large number of poisonous plants that can affect exotic and wild animals. Most often, diagnosis of intoxication from a poisonous plant depends on a history of consumption and the occurrence of compatible clinical signs. There are relatively few analytic tests for the wide diversity of potentially toxic chemicals in plants. Careful examination of GI contents to identify plant fragments is often essential for establishing evidence of consumption. If plant fragments are too small for unaided visual identification, microscopic identification is possible. In such cases, obtaining samples for plants in the environment of the animal for comparison is important. Diagnostic laboratories can often enlist plant experts to assist in plant identification.

Veterinary and human medications

The wide variety of chemicals in this category makes generalization most difficult. If a particular drug is of interest, it is always a good idea to check with the laboratory first. Frequently, toxicology laboratories receive requests for tissue analyses to determine the presence of tranquilizers, anesthesia, or euthanasia agents. Although many can be detected in tissue or fluid samples (eg, whole blood, serum, plasma, or urine), interpretation of results is often impossible because of lack of information relating tissue concentrations with particular adverse sequelae. Interpretation, therefore, is often limited to confirmation of exposure. The most common mistake with regard to submission of samples for drug analysis is the failure to submit a variety of samples, including serum, urine, liver, and kidney (obviously, the latter two postmortem). Depending on the pharmacokinetics of a particular drug and the timing of sample collection, it may be possible to detect the drug in only one or a few of the submitted samples. Chemicals can often be detected in urine samples but not in corresponding serum or plasma samples. The majority of drug testing is for the parent compound; testing for drug metabolites is not as common.

Interpretation of results

As indicated above, all of the information regarding the case is important for proper interpretation of the analytic results. Unfortunately, detected amounts of a toxicant in submitted samples may not provide a definitive answer. Other information, including the time frame and magnitude of exposure, clinical signs, clinical pathologic measurements, gross and histologic examination, and adjunctive testing such as cholinesterase determinations can all be critical to a diagnosis. Often it is impossible to interpret a given tissue concentration because data are not available correlating these with specific adverse effects. In such situations, the diagnostician can only use such phrases as "compatible with toxicosis" or "laboratory results indicate exposure to."

Summary

The increasing sophistication of toxicologic analyses offered by veterinary diagnostic laboratories provides the practitioner with a valuable resource for the diagnosis of exotic and wild animal toxicoses. The availability of such testing is a valuable service that can be offered to veterinary clientele. Appropriate and timely toxicologic testing may permit more successful treatment of affected patients and protect animals and humans from hazardous exposure that might occur if a responsible toxicant goes unrecognized. Perhaps the most critical point to keep in mind, however, is that no matter how sophisticated the toxicologic laboratory, a correct diagnosis is dependent upon the submission of appropriate biologic and environmental samples and interpretation of results based upon the best available historical and scientific information.

References

[1] Fitzgerald KT. Taking a toxicologic history. In: Peterson ME, Talcott PA, editors. Small animal toxicology. 2nd edition. St. Louis (MO): Elsevier Saunders; 2006. p. 38–44.
[2] Volmer PA, Meerdinck GL. Diagnostic toxicology for the small animal practitioner. Vet Clin North Am Small Anim Pract 2002;32:357–65.
[3] Osweiler GD. Diagnostic toxicology. In: Osweiler GD, editor. The national veterinary medical series. Toxicology. Philadephia: Williams and Wilkins; 1996. p. 37–46.
[4] Poppenga RH, Braselton WE Jr. Effective use of analytical laboratories for the diagnosis of toxicologic problems in small animal practice. Vet Clin North Am Small Anim Pract 1990;20: 293–306.
[5] Fitzgerald KT. Establishing a minimum database in small animal poisoning. In: Peterson ME, Talcott PA, editors. Small animal toxicology. 2nd edition. St. Louis (MO): Elsevier Saunders; 2006. p. 60–72.
[6] Minnick PD, Braselton WE, Meerdinck GL, et al. Altered serum element concentrations due to laboratory usage of Vacutainer tubes. Vet Hum Toxicol 1982;24:413–4.
[7] Rosenthal KL, Johnston MS, Shofer FS, et al. Psittacine plasma concentrations of elements: daily fluctuations and clinical implications. J Vet Diagn Invest 2005;17:239–44.

VETERINARY
CLINICS
Exotic Animal Practice

Vet Clin Exot Anim 11 (2008) 211–228

Emergency Care and Managing Toxicoses in the Exotic Animal Patient

Marla Lichtenberger, DVM, DACVECC[a,b,*], Jill A. Richardson, DVM[c,d]

[a]11015 North Mequon Square Drive, Mequon, WI 53092, USA
[b]Milwaukee Emergency Clinic for Animals and Specialty Services, Milwaukee, WI, USA
[c]The Hartz Mountain Corporation, 400 Plaza Drive, Secaucus, NJ 07094, USA
[d]Veterinary Information Network, PO Box 3121, Secaucus, NJ 07096, USA

The poisoned exotic veterinary patient remains a significant challenge to the clinician. A patient presenting with the history of exposure to a toxin or poison should be considered to have a potentially life-threatening problem. The clinician faced with a critical patient must immediately evaluate the need for lifesaving procedures and support. As always, the emergent patient is examined and treated using the ABCs (airway, breathing, circulation). Resuscitation with establishment of the airway, adequate support of ventilation and perfusion, and maintenance of all vital signs (including heart rate, blood pressure, capillary refill time, color of mucous membranes, and temperature) must be accomplished first. Continuous cardiac and pulse oximetry monitoring is essential. Maintenance of blood pressure, tissue perfusion, and acid-base disturbance may require adequate volume replacement. In addition to basic airway management, some patients may require advanced management that includes endotracheal intubation. Intubation offers the advantages of complete airway control, protecting the patient from aspiration of gastric contents, providing a route for suctioning of secretions, and optimizing both oxygenation and ventilation. The first part of this article details the ABCs of emergency medicine including fluid therapy.

Poisonings and intoxications often affect the patient's level of consciousness or result in hyperactivity. Affected patients may show alterations of consciousness that range from seizures to coma. Numerous drugs and chemicals may result in hyperactivity, restlessness, pacing, tremors, or apparent hallucinations. Severe prolonged hyperactivity may result in hyperthermia

* Corresponding author.
E-mail address: marlavet@aol.com (M. Lichtenberger).

1094-9194/08/$ - see front matter © 2008 Elsevier Inc. All rights reserved.
doi:10.1016/j.cvex.2008.01.002 *vetexotic.theclinics.com*

and exhaustion. The principles of neurologic management are relatively straightforward and are discussed in this article.

The last part of the article provides the clinician with guidelines for decontamination and critical care management of some of the more common toxicoses in exotic animals.

ABCs of emergency medicine

Airway

Lifesaving interventions begin with the airway. Many poisons directly or indirectly cause fluid or secretions to build up in the airway. These may occlude the airway leading to hypoxic complications and possibly even death.

Evaluate the airway by direct visualization if possible. Patients that are awake and alert are not likely to need airway intervention, but the clinician should be alert for signs of deterioration that can result in rapid loss of airway control. Loud upper airway sounds such as gurgling or stridor are indications of a patient with an upper airway obstruction. Patients that are comatose or obtunded may lack a protective gag reflex and may be in danger of rapidly losing their airway. If any doubt exists regarding a patient's ability to protect the airway, endotracheal intubation should be performed. Tracheal intubation (tracheostomy, tracheotomy) is necessary when endotracheal intubation is not possible because of physical obstruction of the rostral trachea.

Breathing

Once the airway is determined to be open and secure, an evaluation of breathing must be performed. Respiratory complications fall into the categories of hypoxia (PaO_2 < 60 Torr using arterial blood gas determination or SpO_2 < 90% using a pulse oximeter to obtain hemoglobin saturation) or ventilatory failure ($PaCo_2$ > 60 Torr). If there is evidence of hypoxia (SpO_2 < 90%), provide supplemental oxygen (see the following section) and observe response. If there is no response to supplemental oxygen (SpO_2 remains < 90%), begin assisted ventilation (see later in this article). If the PaO_2 is greater than 60 Torr, begin immediate assisted ventilation.

Supplemental oxygen treatment
1. Facemask using an anesthesia machine as an oxygen source.
2. Blow-by oxygen administration using an oxygen line or mask in front of the patient's face and set at a high flow rate (inspiratory rate of approximately 5 L/min for every 5 kg body weight).
3. Oxygen bag using a clear plastic bag over the head or body and placing the oxygen line inside. Initial flow rates of oxygen must be rapid enough to inflate the bag, but may be slowed to 100 to 200 mL/kg/min as maintenance.
4. Nasal catheter is one of the most efficient, economical routes of oxygen supplementation. The flow rate is usually maintained at 50 mL/kg/min.

5. Oxygen hood can be provided with the help of an Elizabethan collar. The end of the collar is covered with saran wrap so that it covers 75% of the opening to let exhaled gases escape.
6. Oxygen cage can be used according to the manufacturer's recommendations for flow rates.
7. Air sac intubation in the case of a bird [1].

Assisted ventilation

Ventilation may be provided with the use of an endotracheal tube or tracheal tube. The patient should be ventilated using a tidal volume of 10 to 12 mL/kg and rate of 12 breaths per minute. In case of an emergency, a commercial bag-valve device (Ambu-bag; Ridge Medical, Lombard, IL) is available for temporary ventilation. The oxygen line can be hooked directly to the Ambu-bag.

Circulation

Many poisoned or intoxicated patients are presented in a state of cardiovascular collapse that must be recognized and treated early in the course of events after (or in conjunction with) airway and breathing assessment and treatment.

Assessment

1. Check pulse rate and rhythm. Ausculte heart rate and rhythm. Start cardiopulmonary-cerebral resuscitation (CPCR) if there is no pulse or heart beat (see CPCR in the next section).
2. Assess pulse quality using the femoral artery on the medial side of the rear limb or medial ulnar vein in the bird. If the pulse is easily palpated, the systolic blood pressure is likely higher than 80 mm Hg.
3. Check systolic indirect Doppler blood pressure with the target pressure being higher than 90 mm Hg in all species. In the poisoned patient, hypotension is usually due to hypovolemia secondary to vomiting, diarrhea, or blood loss (see treatment for hypovolemic hypotension later in this article). Hypotension can also be due to vasodilatation (eg, venodilatation and/or arteriolar dilatation) or decreased cardiac output (eg, dysrhythmias, decreased contractility).
4. Assess mucous membrane color (normal color is pink) and capillary refill time (CRT; 1 to 2 seconds is normal and expect pale pink or white mucous membranes with hypotension).

Treatment for CPCR

In veterinary medicine, basic life support is performed based on the ABC approach. After establishing a patent airway and placing an endotracheal tube, positive pressure ventilation with 100% oxygen should be initiated.

Intubation is easily performed in the ferret and bird, whereas in the rabbit and other small mammals it is more difficult to perform this procedure. If endotracheal intubation can not be accomplished after the first attempt, then consider placing a tight fitting mask with forced ventilations. The other alternative is to perform a tracheostomy [2]. Ventilate with 100% oxygen at 20 to 30 times per minute (ie, traditional ratio of chest compressions to lung inflations is 5:1). This can be administered either via an Ambu-bag connected to an oxygen tube, or via an anesthesia machine.

Circulation involves closed-chest cardiac massage. The primary goal of circulatory support is to supply adequate blood flow to essential organs, specifically the heart and the brain. When external chest compressions are used, blood flow in small mammals as in cats is produced by the cardiac pump theory (ie, direct pressure applied over the heart leads to compression of the myocardium and increased cardiac output). The thoracic pump theory, which is important for animals weighing more than 7 kg, uses the increase in overall intrathoracic pressure to cause filling and forward flow of blood into the heart. Birds have a keel and no diaphragm and therefore direct heart compression nor the thoracic pump theory will apply. CPCR in birds will be discussed separately.

The chest compressions of 80 to 100 times per minute directly compress the myocardium, which leads to increased cardiac output. It is important that both hands be placed on each side of the chest with compressions done at the widest portion of the chest. The duration of the compression should take up half of the total compression-release cycle. The team should continually assess its efforts at CPR. Check to see if the efforts are generating a palpable pulse. If no pulse is felt, increase the force of chest compressions and assess the electrocardiogram. Different cardiac arrhythmias may require specific treatments (see Fig. 1).

Treatment for hypovolemic hypotension
Fluid therapy for the avian patient. Any sick, debilitated bird presenting for emergency care should immediately be placed in a warm incubator (temperature at 85 to 90°F [29.4 to 32.1°C]) with oxygen supplementation for 8 to 12 hours. When active external hemorrhage is present, this must be stopped immediately. Most birds benefit from the administration of warmed crystalloids at 3 mL/100 g body weight intravenously (IV), intraosseously (IO), or subcutaneously (SQ). Birds should be offered food and water during this time. When the bird appears stable (alert, responsive) and can be safely anesthetized with mask isoflurane (Abbott Laboratory, North Chicago, IL) or sevoflurane (Abbott Laboratory), diagnostics and treatment or hypovolemia and dehydration can be performed. Blood pressure monitoring using an indirect Doppler blood pressure monitor and an electrocardiogram (ECG) should be used during these procedures. External heat should be provided during these procedures, using a heating pad or forced warm heating blanket.

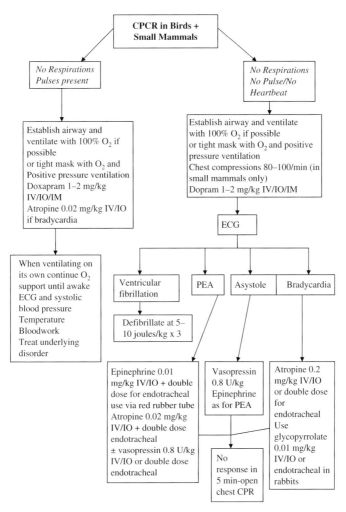

Fig. 1. CPCR in birds and small mammals. Follow the chart for treatment protocol for respiratory and/or cardiac arrest.

The Doppler cuff can be placed on the distal humerus or femur and Doppler probe on the medial surface of the proximal ulna or tibiotarsus respectively. The blood pressure of various avian species under isoflurane or sevoflurane anesthesia at the author's clinic (Lichtenberger) is 90 to 140 mm Hg systolic. When blood pressures are below 90 mm Hg systolic, birds are treated for hypovolemia (when hypotension is the result of hypovolemia as in vomiting, diarrhea, or blood loss) as given below. Bolus administration of crystalloids (10 mL/kg) and colloids (hetastarch 6% or oxyglobin at 5 mL/kg) can be given IV or IO until blood pressure is greater than 90 mm Hg systolic. In the author's experience (Lichtenberger), one or two bolus infusions are usually required. Blood pressure monitoring helps the veterinarian identify cardiovascular problems in patients under anesthesia earlier than when using an ECG only. Immediate correction of hypotension (systolic blood pressure less than 90 mm Hg) with a fluid bolus will help correct hypovolemia and prevent cardiovascular collapse and death.

Isotonic crystalloids at 15 mL/kg (ie, lactated ringers solution, plasma-lyte, normasol) together with colloids at 5 mL/kg (hetastarch or oxyglobin) are bloused intraosseously or intravenously until the indirect Doppler systolic blood pressure is greater than 90 mm Hg.

The use of hypertonic solutions has gained popularity. Hypertonic saline is also a crystalloid, but it has the advantage of restoring vascular volume rapidly by osmotically drawing water from the interstitium to the intravascular space. Small volumes of 7.5% saline can be given at 3 mL/kg together with hetastarch at 5 mL/kg as a slow bolus once. If the systolic blood pressure remains below 90 mm Hg, continued boluses of isotonic crystalloids and colloids are continued until the systolic blood pressure is greater than 90 mm Hg.

Fluid therapy for the small mammal. The blood volume in the ferret and rabbit is 50 to 60 mL/kg, in contrast to 90 mL/kg in the dog. When intravascular volume deficits result in poor perfusion, it has been recommended in the past that crystalloids be administered fast in volumes equivalent to the animal's blood volume. However, resuscitation with crystalloids alone can result in significant pulmonary and pleural fluid accumulation. The resultant hypoxemia contributes to the shock pathophysiology. Rabbits, ferrets, and small mammals are difficult to resuscitate from hypotensive episodes. In the rabbit, when baroreceptors have detected inadequate arterial stretch, it has been found that vagal fibers are stimulated simultaneously with sympathetic fibers. As a result, the heart rate may be normal or slow, instead of the typical tachycardia demonstrated by the dog. This baroreceptor response may be similar in the ferret and other small mammals. In the authors' experience, normal ferrets and rabbits have heart rates between 180 and 240 beats per minute (bpm), systolic blood pressure between 90 and 120 mm Hg, and temperatures between 100 and 102°F (37.7 to 38.8°C). Most ferrets, rabbits, and small mammals presented for hypovolemic shock demonstrate heart rates less than 200 bpm, hypotension (systolic blood pressure less than 90 mm Hg), and hypothermia (temperature < 98°F [36.6°C]). Because cardiac output is a function of contractility and rate, the compensatory response to shock normally seen in dogs and birds is most likely blunted in ferrets, rabbits, and small mammals.

The hyperdynamic signs of shock seen in the dog and birds are not typically seen in the cat, ferret, rabbit, and small mammals. Shock in the cat, rabbit, ferret, and small mammal is most commonly decompensatory, manifested by normal or bradycardia (heart rate <180 bpm), hypothermia (<98°F or 36.6°C), weak or nonpalpable pulses with hypotension, and profound mental depression. The mucous membranes are gray or white and capillary refill is not evident. The bradycardia and low cardiac output contribute to hypothermia, and hypothermia accentuates the bradycardia.

Resuscitation from hypovolemic shock can be safely accomplished with a combination of crystalloids and colloids and rewarming procedures. In the hypovolemic ferret, rabbit, and small mammal, a rapid infusion of isotonic crystalloids is administered at 10 to 15 mL/kg. Hetastarch is administered at 5 mL/kg over 5 to 10 minutes. The blood pressure is checked, and once it is above 40 mm Hg systolic, then only maintenance crystalloids are given while the patient is aggressively warmed. The warming should be done within the next 30 minutes to 1 hour with warm water bottles and warming the IV fluids. IV fluid warmers facilitate core temperature warming (Elltec Warmel WL-1, Gaymar Industries Inc, Oakland Park, NY). Once the animal's rectal temperature has risen to 99°F, the blood pressure is rechecked. Once the rectal temperature approaches 98°F, it appears that the adrenergic receptors begin to respond to catecholamines and fluid therapy. Temperatures during this rewarming phase must be checked frequently in all exotic species to prevent hyperthermia.

The hetastarch can then be repeated at 5-mL/kg increments over 15 minutes until the systolic blood pressure rises above 90 mm Hg (systolic). Most commonly, no further resuscitation fluids are required. The use of 7.5% hypertonic saline at 3 mL/kg with hetastarch at 3 mL/kg as a slow bolus over 10 to 15 minutes can be used once to increase as an initial bolus. The rectal temperature must be maintained as needed by a warm incubator and warmed fluids. If the indirect systolic Doppler blood pressure does not increase to greater than 90 mm Hg, another 5 mL/kg of hetastarch may be required followed by a constant rate infusion of hetastarch at 3 to 5 mL/kg/h. If endpoint parameters (normal blood pressure, heart rate, mucous membrane color, and CRT) are still not obtained, the animal is evaluated and treated for causes of nonresponsive shock (ie, excessive vasodilation or vasoconstriction, hypoglycemia, electrolyte imbalances, acid-base disorder, cardiac dysfunction, hypoxemia). If cardiac function is normal, and glucose, acid-base, and electrolyte abnormalities have been corrected, treatment for nonresponsive shock is continued. Oxyglobin has not been approved for use in the cat, ferret, rabbit, or small mammal, but has been used successfully at our hospital when given in small-volume boluses. Titrate 2 mL/kg boluses given over 10 to 15 minutes until normal heart rate and blood pressure (systolic blood pressure greater than 90 mm Hg) are obtained. This is followed by a continuous rate infusion of oxyglobin at 0.2 to 0.4 mL/kg/h.

Consciousness

Poisonings and intoxication often affect the patient's level of consciousness. Affected patients may show alterations of consciousness, pupils, ocular movements, and motor function. Affected patients may show alterations of consciousness that range from seizures to coma.

Assessment

Repeated assessment every 15 minutes is essential during the initial 2 hours after presentation. Any signs of worsening (given below in the neurological exam signs) should be treated as described in the section on stupor and coma.

Level of consciousness

Consciousness is defined as an awareness of self and the environment. The different states from normal to worse include alert, depressed, agitated, stuporous, and coma. Any change in consciousness to a worse sign will require treatment (given below in the neurological exam signs).

Pupils

Midpoint fixed pupils or a unilateral or bilateral dilated pupil suggests structural lesion of the midbrain and a guarded prognosis. Pinpoint pupils indicate a lesion of the cerebrum. Treatment is recommended when the pupils change from pinpoint to dilated or fixed.

Ocular movements

A disturbance of normal ocular movements as loss of doll's eyes movements (normal lateral rotation with a fast phase and slow-phase nystagmus) suggests structural disease and a guarded prognosis.

Seizures

Seizures remain one of the most common complications resulting from poisoning or intoxications. Seizures can result in hyperthermia, neurogenic pulmonary edema, or aspiration pneumonia.

Treatment involves maintaining an open, secure airway with an endotracheal tube if necessary and assisted ventilation. Benzodiazepines (midazolam) can be given at 0.25 to 0.50 mg/kg intravenously or intramuscularly. If the seizures are not controlled or recur, a phenobarbital load is recommended using phenobarbital at 4 mg/kg intravenously or intramuscularly for 2 doses given 20 minutes apart. Always check blood glucose and calcium and replace if necessary. Check the temperature and if hyperthermic use cool fluids to reduce the temperature.

Agitation

Numerous drugs and chemicals (most common are amphetamines, antihistamines, baclofen, cocaine, lead, marijuana, pseudoephedrine) may result in hyperactivity that is not under control of the patient.

Treatment involves administration of midazolam (0.25 to 0.50 mg/kg IM or IV). Place an IV or IO catheter and treat hyperthermia, if present, with cool fluids, and hypoglycemia with dextrose. Tremors are treated with a muscle relaxer (methocarbamol at 50 to 100 mg/kg as needed and not to exceed 500 mg/kg/day).

Stupor or coma

Numerous toxins reduce the level of consciousness directly by depressing the brain's reticular activating system. Stupor (aroused with a noxious stimulus) or coma (not aroused with a noxious stimulus) may also be a postictal sign following a toxin-induced seizure.

Treatment is started with the initial resuscitation of the cardiopulmonary system in case of cardiac or respiratory arrest (see Fig. 1). An IV or IO catheter is placed and hypotension can be treated using 7.5% hypertonic saline (3 mL/kg IV or IO) as a slow bolus over 10 to 15 minutes followed by hetastarch slow bolus (3 to 5 mL/kg). Indirect systolic Doppler blood pressure is rechecked and if lower than 90 mm Hg, then repeated bolus of hetastarch is given until systolic indirect blood pressure is higher than 90 mm Hg. The patient can be continued on 0.9% saline at the maintenance rate. If the patient deteriorates (see assessment of neurologic signs) but the blood pressure is normal, the above treatment using hypertonic saline and hetastarch is given. Any signs of agitation should be treated using butorphanol IM or IV at 0.4 to 0.6 mg/kg (1 to 2 mg/kg IM, IV, or IO in birds).

Decontamination and managing toxicoses in pet birds and small mammals

Even exotic animals are exposed to commonly found items in the home that can potentially be dangerous. However, reports of toxicoses in pet birds and in small mammals are not as high a volume as those reported in dogs and cats. Since most pet birds and small mammals limited activity outside their cages, toxicoses are not commonly noted. However, problems may arise and with prompt and proper treatment, some situations may be reversed for the better. Just like with dogs and cats, stabilization and supportive care are critical for full recovery of the exotic patient. Many situations involving potentially toxic agents can be avoided simply by providing client education about household dangers. This section's purpose is to address decontamination and the management of the most common types of toxicant exposures in pet birds and small mammals.

Decontamination guidelines

Preventing absorption of the substance through decontamination is an important step in treating a toxicosis.

Dermal exposures

With light dermal exposures, the pet can be gently spritzed with a solution of mild liquid dishwashing detergent and warm water, softly rubbed, and then spritzed with plain warm water to remove soap. With small-sized small mammals, it may be easier to gently wipe the animal off with a warm wet washcloth. This process should be performed in a gentle manner and can be repeated as needed.

A more thorough bathing would be needed with heavy exposures. Multiple warm baths may be needed with sticky substances. Following the bath, the patient should be lightly dried, kept warm, and monitored for signs of hypothermia. Bathing is contraindicated if the animal is seriously ill; always stabilize the patient first. With corrosive or irritating substances, the animal's skin should be monitored for redness, swelling, or pain.

Ocular exposures

With ocular exposures, the animal's eyes should be gently flushed with tepid tap water or with physiologic saline. The use of an eyedropper to gently administer the flush is recommended in birds and small mammals. Fluorescein staining and follow-up examinations are warranted with exposures to corrosive agents or if clinical signs of redness, pain, or ocular discharge occur.

Oral exposures

Dilution with milk, nonacidic juicy fruits, water or demulcents is recommended in cases of corrosive or irritating substance ingestion. Close monitoring of the oral cavity is recommended following ingestion of corrosive agents, as they may lead to tissue damage, necrosis, or inflammation of the mouth, esophagus, and stomach or crop.

Emesis is most productive if performed within 2 to 3 hours postingestion. Dogs, cats, ferrets, and potbelly pigs are examples of house pets that can vomit. Emetics should not be given to rodents, rabbits, birds, horses, and ruminants. Feeding a small moist meal before inducing vomiting can increase chances of an adequate emesis. Emetics generally empty 40% to 60% of the stomach contents and are assumed to be more beneficial than gastric lavages. Emesis is contraindicated with ingestion of alkalis, acids, corrosive agents, or hydrocarbons. The preexisting condition of the animal also determines the indication for using an emetic. Emesis should not be induced in an animal that has a history of epilepsy, cardiovascular disease, or is debilitated. Emesis should not be attempted if the animal has already vomited, or is exhibiting signs of severe stimulation or severe lethargy.

Activated charcoal is considered a nonspecific adsorbent that binds to many substances through weak forces, and prevents their systemic absorption. It is not an effective adsorbent for corrosive substances, petroleum distillates, or heavy metals [3–5]. Activated charcoal can be given to birds with a dosing syringe, an eyedropper, or lavage tube, although extreme caution must be used to avoid aspiration. Dosage of activated charcoal in most species is 1 g/kg (or 1 to 3 mg/g body weight) [4,5].

Cathartics are substances that enhance the elimination of activated charcoal, but should be used cautiously in birds and small mammals. Cathartics can be added to solutions of activated charcoal, or premixed combinations are available. Never use cathartics when the patient is dehydrated. Bulking agents can be useful in removing small solid objects from the animal's gastrointestinal tract, such as lead paint chips. One-half teaspoon of psyllium mixed with 60 cc baby food gruel has been suggested as a bulking agent for birds and small mammals and can be administered with a dosing syringe or eyedropper [6]. Use extreme caution to avoid aspiration. The mixture may be repeated to ensure complete removal of the objects. Peanut butter has also been recommended as a bulking agent.

During decontamination, the animal should be continuously monitored. Routinely evaluate vital signs, and the parameters most likely to be affected. Preventive measures such as gastric protection or antibiotics may be needed. Additional measures, such as nutritional and hydration support, are key components for full recovery. Good nursing care should be given until the animal completely recovers.

Gastric (or crop) lavage should not be performed in cases of caustic or petroleum distillate ingestion. General anesthesia should be performed when performing a lavage.

Common household toxicants

Poisonous plants

The following is a partial list of plants that have been shown to cause toxicity in dogs and cats. The severity of signs or toxicity of these plants in small mammals or birds has not been thoroughly studied.

Potentially cardiotoxic plants
    Lily of the Valley (*Convallaria majalis*)
    Oleander (*Nerium oleander*)
    Rhododendron species
    Japanese, American, English, and Western Yew (*Taxus* species)
    Foxglove (*Digitalis purpurea*)
    Kalanchoe species
    Kalmia species

Plants that could cause kidney failure
    Rhubarb (*Rheum* species), leaves only
    Lilies, all parts, only reported in cats

Plants that could cause liver failure
    Cycad, Sago, Zamia Palm (*Cycad* species)
    Amanita mushrooms

Plants that can cause multisystem effects
    Autumn crocus (*Colchicum* species)
    Castor bean (*Ricinus* species)

Plants containing calcium oxalate crystals

Peace lilies, Calla lilies, Philodendrons, Dumb cane, and Mother-in-law, and Pothos plants contain insoluble calcium oxalate crystals. These crystals can cause mechanical irritation of the oral cavity and tongue of birds when plant material is ingested. Clinical signs that are usually include regurgitation, oral pain, dysphagia, and anorexia. The signs are rarely severe and usually respond to supportive care.

Peace lilies (*Spathiphyllum* species)
Calla lily (*Zantedeschia aethiopiea*)
Philodendron (*Philodendron* species)
Dumb cane (*Dieffenbachia* species)
Mother-in-law plant (*Monstera* species)
Pothos (*Epipremnum* species)

Avocado (Persea americana)

The toxic principle in avocado is persin. Leaves, fruit, bark, and seeds of the avocado have been reported to be toxic to birds, rabbits, guinea pigs, and various other species. Clinical effects seen with avocado toxicoses include respiratory distress, generalized congestion, hydropericardium, anasarca, and death. Onset of clinical signs usually occurs after 12 hours of ingestion with death occurring within 1 to 2 days of the time of exposure. Treatment for recent avocado ingestion includes decontamination via crop lavage and activated charcoal; bulking diets may help prevent absorption. Close monitoring for cardiovascular and pulmonary signs should follow. Treatment with humidified oxygen and minimal handling may be required with dyspneic animals; diuretics may be helpful with pulmonary edema [6].

Heavy metals

Zinc

Sources of zinc include hardware such as wire, screws, bolts and nuts, and US pennies. Pennies minted since 1983 contain 99.2% zinc and 0.8% copper and one penny contains approximately 2440 mg of elemental zinc [6–9]. The process of galvanization involves the coating of wire or other material like food or water bowls with a zinc-based compound to prevent rust. Zinc toxicosis can affect the renal, hepatic, and hematopoietic tissues. Clinical signs of zinc toxicoses in birds may include polyuria, polydipsia, diarrhea, weight loss, weakness, anemia, cyanosis, seizures, and death [6,7]. In mammals, clinical signs of toxicoses include hemolytic anemia, vomiting (in species that can vomit), abdominal pain, and weakness.

In regard to diagnosis, radiography of the abdomen may reveal the presence of metallic objects in the gastrointestinal tract. Serum zinc levels may be obtained using blood collected from plastic syringes (no rubber grommets) and stored in Royal blue top vaccutainers to minimize contamination with exogenous zinc [6–8]. The pancreas is considered to be the best tissue for postmortem zinc analysis [6].

The key to treatment is the removal the sources of zinc from the gastro-intestinal tract through endoscopy or gastrotomy/enterotomy. The success of the removal process can be assessed with radiographs. Activated charcoal is not indicated with zinc exposures [6,8]. Bulk cathartics, such as psyllium, peanut butter, mineral oil, and corn oil may aid in the removal of zinc objects from the gastrointestinal tract. The use of chelators may not be necessary in cases where prompt removal of the zinc source is accomplished [6,8]. If chelation therapy is instituted, careful monitoring of renal parameters is important for the duration of therapy. In addition, treatment for symptomatic animals should include blood replacement therapy, as needed parenteral fluids, and good nursing care such as forced feeding or hand feeding.

Lead

Sources of lead include paint, toys, drapery weights, linoleum, batteries, plumbing materials, galvanized wire, solder, stained glass, fishing sinkers, lead shot, foil from champagne bottles, and improperly glazed bowls [6,8]. Lead affects multiple tissues, especially the gastrointestinal tract and renal, hematopoietic, and nervous systems. Lead combines with erythrocytes in circulating blood increasing red blood cell fragility, anemia, and capillary damage. It can also cause segmental demyelination of neurons and necrosis of renal tubular epithelium, gastrointestinal tract mucosa, and liver parenchyma. Clinical signs seen in psittacine birds are often vague and may include lethargy, weakness, anorexia, regurgitation, polyuria, ataxia, circling, and convulsions [6].

Diagnosis of lead poisoning includes radiography of the abdomen, which may reveal evidence of metal in the ventriculus. Blood levels of lead are helpful to confirm lead toxicoses in animals with suspicious radiographic changes [6,8]. Removal of lead particles via bulk diet therapy, endoscopy, or surgery is recommended [10–20]. Succimer and Ca EDTA are both considered to be effective chelating agents [6,8]. In addition, good supportive care, including seizure control, is recommended until full recovery.

Inhalants in pet birds

The avian respiratory tract is extremely sensitive to inhalant irritants. Any strong odor or smoke could be potentially toxic [6,7]. Polytetrafluoroethylene (PTFE)-coated cookware or cooking utensils can emit toxic fumes when overheated ($>280°F$) [6,7]. Clinical signs may include acute death, rales, dyspnea, ataxia, depression, and restless behavior [10,21]. Hemorrhage and edema in pulmonary tissues leads to respiratory failure and death. Prognosis is usually guarded to poor. Treatment for inhalation toxicoses includes the administration of oxygen, rapidly acting corticosteroids, diuretics, analgesics, parenteral antibiotics, and topical ophthalmic antibiotic ointment [6].

A bronchodilator may be needed for bronchospasms. In most cases, prognosis is guarded to poor.

Rodenticides

Anticoagulant rodenticides

Anticoagulant rodenticides are divided into two classifications: short acting (warfarin) and long acting (pindone, diphacinone, difethialone, chlorophacinone, brodifacoum, and bromadiolone). Anticoagulant rodenticides act through competitive inhibition of vitamin K epoxide reductase, which halts the recycling of vitamin K. Factor VII it is the first parameter affected. It is located in the extrinsic pathway, and can be measured with prothrombin time (PT). In early cases of toxicoses, the PT when checked between 36 and 72 hours will be elevated, but the animal will still appear clinically normal [8]. Beyond 72 hours, factor IX becomes depleted, and shuts down the intrinsic pathway at which time hemorrhage is a possible effect. The presence of circulating clotting factors in normal animals is the reason for the delay in the development of signs. Clinical signs of an anticoagulant poisoning are seen several days postexposure and include hemorrhage, pale mucous membranes, weakness, exercise intolerance, lameness, dypsnea, coughing, and swollen joints [8,9].

As for diagnostics, the PT test will confirm the presence of the extrinsic and common pathways. It will be elevated with any deficiency of factor VII, and is the best test for early detection (due to the short half-life of factor VII) of a vitamin K–impaired coagulopathy. Recent vitamin K_1 administration could result in misleading PT values because new clotting factor synthesis only requires 6 to 12 hours. PIVKA (proteins induced by vitamin K absence or antagonists) detects a build up of nonfunctional clotting factor precursors. With a depletion of vitamin K, a build up of clotting factor precursors occurs. Normal animals do not have PIVKA present in the circulation.

Decontamination is only effective with recent exposures in asymptomatic animals. Treating an animal with overt anticoagulant poisoning begins with stabilization of the animal. Transfusions with whole blood or plasma may be necessary to replace clotting factors. When small mammals are exposed to anticoagulants, it is advised to initiate vitamin K_1 therapy instead of monitoring clotting times [8]. The reason for this would be that even a small dose would probably be one that would cause coagulopathy. Vitamin K_1 should be administered at a dose of 3 to 5 mg/kg/day orally [8]. This dose should be divided and given twice a day or three times a day and should be given with a fatty meal (peanut butter) to enhance absorption [8]. Vitamin K_1 therapy should be given for an extensive amount of time. For example, warfarin can cause effects for about 2 weeks, bromadiolone for about 3 weeks, and the others may cause problems for over 30 days. Vitamin K_1 should never be given intravenously and it is possible to have an anaphylactic reaction when given subcutaneously; however, the injectable formula can be given to small mammals orally. Also, try to avoid the use of other highly protein-bound drugs during the treatment, and instruct the owner to restrict exercise during this time.

Bromethalin

Bromethalin is an uncoupler of oxidative phosphorylation. Bromethalin causes a reduction of ATP. ATP is necessary to sustain the sodium/potassium ion channel pumps. When the pump mechanism is inhibited, fluid build up occurs, which results in fluid-filled vacuoles between myelin sheaths. This leads to decreased nerve impulse conduction [8].

Clinical signs of bromethalin poisoning could occur within 24 hours or up to 2 weeks and include muscle tremors, seizures, hyperexcitability, forelimb extensor rigidity, ataxia, CNS depression, loss of vocalization, paresis, paralysis, and death [8]. Postmortem lesions include cerebral and spinal cord edema, and a spongy appearance to the cerebellum. Aggressive decontamination is most important but is only effective with early exposures. Repeated doses of activated charcoal are recommended. There is no antidote for bromethalin poisoning and supportive care should be given for clinical signs. Agents such as mannitol, furosemide, and corticosteroids may reduce the cerebral edema [8]. Unfortunately, these drugs were of little benefit in reducing the severity of signs in experimental animals. The prognosis is poor for animals showing severe signs. *Ginkgo biloba* has been used experimentally in rats at a dose of 100 mg/kg, although true benefit is not known [8].

Cholecalciferol

Cholecalciferol (vitamin D3) is metabolized in the liver to calcifediol (25-hydroxycholecalciferol). Calcifediol is then metabolized by the kidney to calcitriol (1,25-dihydroxycholecalciferol). Cholecalciferol increases intestinal absorption of calcium, stimulates bone resorption, and enhances renal tubular reabsorption of calcium [8]. This results in a serum calcium increase, which can lead to acute renal failure, cardiovascular abnormalities, and tissue mineralization. Clinical signs of cholecalciferol poisoning usually have a delay in onset and usually occur 18 to 36 hours postingestion. The most common signs seen with cholecalciferol toxicosis include vomiting, diarrhea, inappetence, depression, polyuria, polydipsia, and cardiac arrhythmia. Renal failure arises from the deposition of calcium in the kidney. Postmortem lesions seen with cholecalciferol toxicoses include elevated total kidney calcium concentrations and diffuse hemorrhages of the gastrointestinal tract [8]. Mineralization and necrosis of gastrointestinal, cardiac, and renal tissues may be seen histologically. Aggressive decontamination is most important but is only effective with early exposures. Repeated doses of activated charcoal are recommended. Obtain a baseline serum calcium and BUN (blood urea nitrogen) immediately postexposure. Monitor serum calcium and BUN every 12 to 24 hours each day for 3 days postexposure. If the calcium level remains normal for 96 hours, no further treatment would be needed. Renal effects should be treated with supportive care including fluid diuresis using normal saline fluids help to decrease tubular reabsorption of calcium. Pamidronate inhibits osteoclastic bone resorption and has been used successfully to treat cholecalciferol poisoning in dogs and cats [8]. Furosemide and prednisone are usually used in conjunction with pamidronate treatment.

Human medications

Acetaminophen

Acetaminophen is a synthetic nonopiate derivative of p-aminophenol. Acetaminophen toxicity can result from a single toxic dose or repeated cumulative dosages, which lead to methemoglobinemia and hepatotoxicity [8]. Clinical signs of acetaminophen toxicity are related to methemoglobinemia and hepatotoxicity. Clinical signs include depression, weakness, tachypnea, dyspnea, cyanosis, icterus, vomiting, methemoglobinemia, hypothermia, facial or paw edema, hepatic necrosis, and death. The objective of treatment in acetaminophen toxicity is to replenish glutathione, convert methemoglobin back to hemoglobin, and prevent or treat hepatic necrosis. N-acetylcysteine (NAC) directly binds with acetaminophen metabolites to enhance elimination and serves as a glutathione precursor [8]. The use of cimetidine in combination with NAC and ascorbic acid has been shown to be more effective than any of the agents alone in preventing acetaminophen-induced hepatotoxicity in studies. Ascorbic acid (vitamin C) provides a reserve system for the reduction of methemoglobin back to hemoglobin. Cimetidine can inhibit the cytochrome p-450 oxidation system in the liver and may be useful in reducing the metabolism of acetaminophen [8]. The patient should be monitored for the presence of methemoglobinemia. In cats, methemoglobin values increase within 2 to 4 hours, followed by Heinz body formation. The liver enzymes should be monitored closely. Laboratory evidence of hepatotoxicity generally develops 24 to 36 hours postingestion.

Ibuprofen

Ibuprofen is a substituted phenylalkanoic acid with nonsteroidal anti-inflammatory, antipyretic, and analgesic properties. According to studies of acute ingestion of ibuprofen in dogs, vomiting, diarrhea, nausea, anorexia, gastric ulceration, and abdominal pain can be seen with doses of 50 to 25 mg/kg. These signs in combination with renal damage can be seen at doses at or above 175 mg/kg. At doses at or above 400 mg/kg, CNS effects such as seizure, ataxia, and coma may occur [8,22]. Cats are considered to be twice as sensitive as dogs because they have a limited glucuronyl-conjugating capacity. Ferrets appear to be even more sensitive to ibuprofen than cats and toxicity has been seen at doses as low as 18 mg/kg [8,22].

Most common signs of ibuprofen toxicoses include anorexia, nausea, vomiting, lethargy, diarrhea, melena, ataxia, polyuria, and polydipsia.

Ferrets may go directly into a coma after ingestion of ibuprofen. Renal effects may not be as obvious in ferrets as they are in dogs and cats. Postmortem lesions associated with ibuprofen toxicoses include perforations, erosion, ulceration, and hemorrhage of the gastrointestinal tract. A retrospective study was conducted of ibuprofen ingestion in ferrets that were reported to the American Society for the Prevention of Cruelty to Animals (ASPCA) Animal Poison Control Center. Data analysis included amount ingested and clinical effects. Of the cases with known exposure amounts, the ingested doses ranged from 18 mg/kg to 1500 mg/kg. Ninety-three percent of the ferrets that had ingested ibuprofen developed neurologic signs, such as depression, coma, ataxia, recumbency, tremors, and weakness [8,22]. In addition, 55.2% had one or more gastrointestinal effects including anorexia, vomiting, retching or gagging, diarrhea, and melena. Polydipsia, polyuria, dysuria, renal failure, weight loss, shallow breathing, metabolic acidosis, dehydration, and hypothermia were also reported. Death was reported in four cases. The lowest known dose associated with death was 220 mg/kg [8,22].

The primary goal of treatment is to prevent or treat gastric ulceration, renal failure, CNS effects, and possibly hepatic effects. Fluid diuresis for 24 to 48 hours is recommended. Peritoneal dialysis may be necessary if unresponsive oliguric or anuric renal failure develops. Misoprostol (Cytotec) may be helpful for treating or preventing gastric ulceration caused by ibuprofen. Sucralfate can be used to bind to erosions and ulcers, and protect them from exposure to gastric acid, bile acids, and pepsin [8,22]. H_2 blockers and/or proton pump inhibitors may also be helpful. Gastric protection is recommended for at least 5 to 7 days. When renal failure is a potential, BUN, creatinine, and urine specific gravity should be monitored closely [8,22]. A baseline level and then rechecks at 36, 48, and 72 hours is recommended. The animal should also be monitored for acidosis and electrolyte shifts during treatment. Symptomatic treatment for gastric signs and renal failure should be provided until the animal fully recovers.

References

[1] Chavez W, Echols MS. Bandaging, endoscopy, and surgery in the emergency avian patient. Vet Clin North Am Exot Anim Pract 2007;10(2):419–36.

[2] Hawkins MG, Graham JE. Emergency and critical care of rodents. Vet Clin North Am Exot Anim Pract 2007;10(2):501–31.

[3] Beasley VR, Dorman D. Management of toxicoses. Vet Clin North Am Small Anim Pract 1990;20(2):307–38.

[4] Beasley VR, et al. A systems affected approach to veterinary toxicology. Urbana (IL): University of Illinois Press; 1999. p. 27–69.

[5] Bratich PM, Buck WB, Haschek WM. Prevention of T-2 toxin-induced morphologic effects in the rat by highly activated charcoal. Archives of Toxicology 1990;64(3):251–3.

[6] Richardson JA. Toxicology. In: Ritchie, Lightfoot, Harrison, editors. Avian medicine: principles and application. Palm Beach (FL): Spix Publishing; 2005.

[7] Richardson JA, Murphy LA, Means C, et al. Management of toxicoses in birds. Exotic DVM 2001;3(1):23–7.

[8] Richardson JA. Managing ferret toxicoses. In: Lewington J, editor. Ferret medicine and surgery. Philadelphia: Elsevier; 2007.

[9] Richardson JA, Balabuszko RA. Management of toxicoses in ferrets. Exotic DVM 2000; 2(4):23–6.

[10] Ritchie BW, Harrison GJ, Harrison LR. Avian medicine: principles and applications. Lake Worth (FL): Wingers Publications; 1994. p. 1030–52.

[11] Haddad LM. Acute poisoning. In: Goldman L, Bennett JC, editors. Cecil textbook of medicine. 21st edition. Philadelphia: W.B. Saunders Co.; 2000. p. 515–22.

[12] Kulig K. Initial management of ingestions of toxic substances. N Engl J Med 1992;326: 1677–81.

[13] Walls RM. Rapid sequence intubation. Ann Emerg Med 1993;22:1008–13.

[14] Feldman BF, Zinkl JG, Jain NC. Schalm's veterinary hematology. Baltimore (MD): Lippincott Williams & Wilkins; 2000.

[15] Jenkins JR. Avian critical care and emergency medicine. In: Altman R, Clubb S, Dorrestein G, et al, editors. Avian medicine and surgery. Philadelphia: WB Saunders Co.; 1997. p. 839–64.

[16] Lichtenberger M, Orcutt C, DeBehnke D, et al. Mortality and response to fluid resuscitation after acute blood loss in mallard ducks (Anas platyrhynnchos). Proceedings of the Association of Avian Veterinarians 2002;65–70.

[17] Lichtenberger M. Avian shock, fluids and cardiopulmonary/cerebral resuscitation. International Conference on Exotics 2005 proceedings. 25–9.

[18] Quesenberry K, Hillyer E. Supportive care and emergency therapy. In: Ritchie BW, Harrison GJ, Harrison LR, editors. Avian medicine: principles and application. Lake Worth (FL): Wingers Publishing, Inc.; 1994. p. 406–7.

[19] Rupley A. Critical care of pet birds. Vet Clin North Am Exot Anim Prac 1998;1(1):11–42.

[20] Sturkie PD. Body fluids: blood. In: Sturkie PD, editor. Avian physiology. 4th edition. New York: Springer-Verlag; 1986. p. 102–29.

[21] Plum F, Posner JB. Diagnosis of stupor and coma. 3rd edition. Philadelphia: F.A. Davis Co.; 1980.

[22] Richardson JA, Balabuszko RA. Ibuprofen ingestion in ferrets: 43 cases. January 1995– March 2000. The Journal of Veterinary Emergency and Critical Care 2001;11(1):53–9.

VETERINARY
CLINICS
Exotic Animal Practice

Vet Clin Exot Anim 11 (2008) 229–259

Pet Bird Toxicity and Related Environmental Concerns

Teresa L. Lightfoot, DVM, DABVP–Avian*,
Julie M. Yeager, DVM

*Department of Avian and Exotic Medicine, Florida Veterinary Specialists,
3000 Busch Lake Boulevard, Tampa, FL 33614, USA*

Avian toxicology is significant on several levels. For the individual bird and its owner, the veterinarian's knowledge of potential toxins and their treatment may be life saving. To occupants of the same environment (be that a household or an ecosystem) identification of potential toxins may halt or prevent illness in other exposed individuals. To the greater community, neighborhood, ecosystem, and planet, identification of a toxin, its source, and its physiologic effects on selected populations may provide information and impetus for change that will benefit the environment and all its inhabitants.

Birds, cats, and dogs historically have served as sentinels for human toxicity in the environment. Birds were used as sentinels for coal miners in the United States and England until the middle of the last century. Dangerous levels of carbon monoxide, methane, and other poisonous gasses would affect sentinel canaries before they affected the miners, thus warning them of a dangerous environment. In Japan in 1956, the erratic behavior of feral and outdoor cats that had consumed mercury-contaminated fish was widely noted and reported. This behavior in cats preceded the recognition of human behavioral abnormalities as a result of mercury ingestion. In northwestern Ontario in the 1970s, a river system was contaminated with mercury from a chloralkali plant. Pet cats became ill when they consumed fish from this contaminated river, thereby serving as inadvertent sentinels for this toxicity. Another example of a toxin for which pets serve as sentinels for human toxicity is asbestos. Mesothelioma is a neoplasia of humans and dogs caused by asbestos exposure. The latency period between asbestos exposure and mesothelioma development in people may be more than 25 years; but in

---

* Corresponding author.
E-mail address: lightfoott@aol.com (T.L. Lightfoot).

doi:10.1016/j.cvex.2008.01.006   *vetexotic.theclinics.com*

dogs it has been shown to average 5 to 7 years. Pet dogs with spontaneous mesothelioma have been used to identify environmental exposures that might increase their owner's risk of developing this neoplasia.

Pets may be sensitive sentinels of lead poisoning in children. In Illinois, the children and the pet dogs of families living in questionable housing conditions were tested for exposure to lead. A strong correlation was found between lead levels in the serum of the dogs and the children.

As our knowledge of avian toxicology increases, so likely will knowledge regarding the interrelationship of toxicity and its sequelae in birds and humans. As practitioners, we need to be aware of these potential links, share our findings with our colleagues, both veterinary and human, and inform owners of potential concerns with human health.

On a larger environmental scale, our wild birds—coastal and pelagic seabirds, raptors, songbirds—are objects of studies that detect dangerous levels of heavy metals, pesticides, and other chemicals in bodies of water and sources of food for both animals and humans. Affects on their health and fecundity are of conservational import, and have great significance for the environment and human health.

Authors' Note: For purposes of this article, the emphasis will be on toxins that are most commonly encountered in pet birds and those that are specific to avian species. The vast number of possible toxins makes a complete listing prohibitive. Although toxicity may not have been reported in birds for various agents, poison control organizations can aid the veterinarian in determining the danger of potential toxins and recommend treatment that has been documented in other species (Box 1 for a list of poison control resources). General recommendations for initial treatment of toxicities based on the route of exposure appear in Fig. 1.

This discussion of avian toxicology addresses toxins at three different confidence levels:

1. Toxins to which birds are known, through controlled studies, to be sensitive.
2. Toxins that are generally poisonous to vertebrate species, and to which empirically birds have been noted to be susceptible, but for which there are no controlled studies in avian species.
3. Anecdotal reports of toxicities in birds.

Airborne/inhalant toxins

Polytetrafluoroethylene

The avian respiratory tract is particularly sensitive to airborne irritants and toxins because of specific anatomic and physiologic features of birds [1]. Polytetrafluoroethylene (PTFE) is one of the most common causes of airborne toxicity encountered in pet avian species. This product is found

Box 1. Poison control contacts

- American Association of Poison Control Centers, 1-800-222-1222
- ASPCA Animal Poison Control Hotline, 888-426-4435 ($45 consultation fee), www.aspca.org/apcc. Web site features lists of toxic and nontoxic plants.
- Toxicity to Pets, Livestock, and Wildlife: Contact Centers for Disease Control and Prevention (CDC), 800-232-4636, http://www.atsdr.cdc.gov/consultations/
- Angell Animal Poison Control Hotline, 1-877-2ANGELL ($55.00 consultation fee)

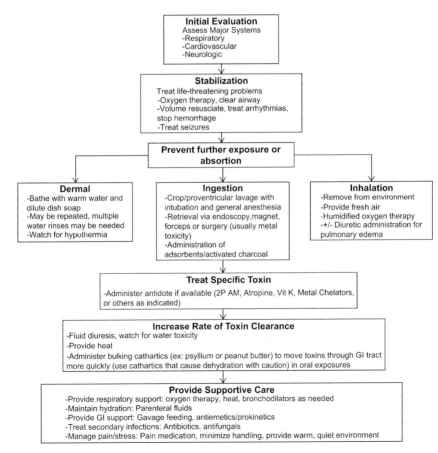

Fig. 1. General approach to treating avian toxicities. Note: This is a general treatment approach. Please refer to specific toxins or consult poison control for more specific treatment.

in nonstick cookware, irons, covers for ironing boards, and heat lamps, among others [2]. When PTFE is heated above 280°C it decomposes into particulates and fluorinated, acidic gasses [3,4] that are toxic when inhaled. Clinical signs may include dyspnea, incoordination, weakness, coma, and death [5]. Pulmonary lesions include severe edema, hemorrhage, and necrosis [3]. Deposition of particulate matter in pulmonary tissues may also be noted on histopathology [3]. Treatment consists of oxygen therapy, bronchodilators, anti-inflammatory drugs, diuretics, antimicrobials to prevent secondary infection, and analgesics. In clinically affected birds, the prognosis is generally poor. Smaller birds such as budgerigars seem to be most sensitive to the effects of PTFE toxicity [1].

Humans may also be affected after exposure to vaporized PTFE products, developing a syndrome called Polymer Fume Fever, which often consists of flu-like symptoms and noncardiogenic pulmonary edema [6–8].

Smoke

Smoke is another source of airborne toxins. Smoke is the general term used for the solid and liquid matter released into the air by combustion (pyrolysis). Exposure to fires, malfunctioning furnaces, engine exhaust, burning food or cooking oil, self-cleaning ovens, or other sources of smoke may induce toxicity [4,5]. Carbon monoxide, hydrogen cyanide, acidic fumes, and particulate matter are components of smoke that cause similar clinical signs to those seen in PTFE toxicity [9]. With smoke inhalation toxicity, dyspnea may not be immediately apparent. It may be several hours before exposed birds demonstrate clinical signs. Smoke inhalation may also lead to immunosuppression and increased susceptibility to infectious disease [10]. In addition to oxygen and bronchodilator therapy, diuretics may be used to treat dyspnea. The efficacy of corticosteroids in the treatment of smoke inhalation is questionable. If used, the duration should be short term, since long-term use of corticosteroids may predispose affected individuals to secondary respiratory infections like aspergillosis [10].

Nicotine

Nicotine in tobacco smoke may be toxic. Birds most likely to be affected are those chronically exposed, usually pets that live in smoking households [11]. One study demonstrated that cotinine, a nicotine metabolite, was significantly higher in the plasma of birds housed in environments with chronic exposure to tobacco smoke than it was in controls. In humans, this metabolite is linked to allergies, asthma, lower respiratory illnesses, and heart disease [12]. Clinical signs in avian patients may include conjunctivitis, rhinitis, other respiratory disease, and dermatitis [4,11,12]. Immediate treatment of severe clinical signs is similar to that of other airborne respiratory toxicities. Long-term treatment is managed by removing the source of smoke from the environment [4,5,11,12]. Second-hand cigarette smoke also releases 1,3-Butadiene vapor, which has been shown to increase atherosclerotic plaques in cockerels. The development of atherosclerosis may be a consideration in birds with a history of prolonged exposure [13]. Ingestion of tobacco products can cause toxicity and clinical signs associated with nicotine consumption, including excitability, gastrointestinal (GI) signs, neurologic signs, and death [4,9]. Nicotine has been shown to interfere with cognitive development in chicks when injected into eggs [14].

Miscellaneous airborne toxins

Other airborne toxins include air fresheners, hair products, nail polish, scented candles, aerosols, gasoline fumes, glues, paints, mothballs, fumigants, and cleaning products such as ammonia or bleach [15]. Sodium hypochlorite (bleach) was shown to cause death within 6 to 12 days in seven birds housed in an aviary that was cleaned with this product. Histopathologic changes included epithelial metaplasia, hyperplasia, deciliation, and ulceration of the trachea [16]. While all inhaled toxins have the potential to cause irritation and damage to the respiratory tract, they may also compromise the immune system. Inhalation of methyl chloride, a chemical compound used as a propellant in aerosol products, has been shown to cause increased susceptibility to respiratory infection in mice [17]. In one author's practice, overheating and melting of a plastic dish in a microwave oven caused the death of a Timneh Gray (*Psittacus erithacus timneh*) within 8 hours of exposure. Histopathologic abnormalities of the lungs were similar to those seen with PTFE toxicity.

Clinical signs and treatment of these toxicities are similar to other airborne toxins. In all cases of potential inhalant toxicity, birds should be removed from the environment as soon as possible after exposure has occurred and placed in a well-ventilated or oxygenated environment [5,15].

Ingested toxins

Heavy metal toxicity

The definition of a heavy metal depends on its usage. In the strict chemical designation, heavy metals are defined as metals that do not normally occur in living organisms (ie, mercury, lead, cadmium) and can cause illness. In a medical context, the term heavy metal generally refers to any metal that is potentially toxic. For this discussion, heavy metals will include those that are required by living organisms in trace amounts, including iron, copper, manganese, and zinc, but which at excessive levels can be detrimental. This discussion does not include the radioactive heavy metals, such as uranium and plutonium.

Heavy metal toxicosis is commonly seen in both pet and wild birds, with lead (Pb) and zinc (Zn) toxicity being the most frequently diagnosed in pet birds [4,5]. Historically, lead was the most common metal toxicity seen in pet

birds. However, in recent years, as lead is used less frequently in home products and knowledge of its toxicity in children has expanded [18], the incidence of lead toxicity (also known as plumbism) in humans and other
animals has decreased [4,19].

Zinc toxicity occurs when zinc-containing items are ingested. Common
sources of avian zinc toxicity include the coating on galvanized wire cages,
galvanized toys, food and water dishes, and hardware (note: the process of
galvanization may include coating with a metal alloy that is more than 98%
zinc and can contain 1% lead). Larger birds may ingest pennies, and those
minted after 1982 have a core containing a high percentage of zinc [4,20].
Clinical signs of zinc toxicity may include lethargy, weakness, polydipsia
and polyuria, diarrhea, regurgitation (particularly passive regurgitation of
water), and less commonly neurologic signs or hemoglobinurea [4,5,15]. Decreased fertility and sudden death were also attributed to zinc ingestion in
a group of orange-bellied parrots housed in galvanized wire caging [21]. A
heterophilia and/or an anemia may be present. Radiographs may demonstrate metal density in the GI tract, usually in the ventriculus; however, it
is possible in zinc toxicities to find no radiographic evidence of metal
[5,22]. Plasma zinc concentrations above 4 parts per million (ppm) are suggestive of toxicosis. Some anecdotal reports suggest that levels as low as
2.5 ppm may be related to clinical disease. A range of 1.25 to 2.29 ppm
was found in clinically normal Hispaniolan Amazon parrots [23]. However,
birds may be clinically affected without high plasma zinc concentrations [5].
One study on the determination of diurnal fluctuations in plasma levels of
several metals, including zinc, indicated that in addition to cyclic fluctuations, the established normal ranges require further study [22]. (Note,
10 µg/dL = 0.1 ppm.) It is important that blood samples be collected in
royal blue top tubes (nonrubber) to prevent contamination of the sample
from zinc found in other rubber stoppers [4,24].

Postmortem diagnosis is best made through analysis of zinc levels in tissue samples of the pancreas, liver, and kidney [25]. Kidney zinc concentrations were found to be 175 ppm in a trumpeter swan (*Cygnus buccinator*)
that died from zinc poisoning [26]. Other histologic changes that may be
seen with zinc heavy metal toxicosis are nonspecific and include loss of
architecture and apoptosis of individual cells as well as zymogen granule depletion of the pancreas [26,27], erosion of the ventriculus [26,27], and acute
tubular necrosis in the kidneys [26].

Lead

Before 1955, house paints in the United States often contained up to 50%
lead. The sweet taste of lead encourages ingestion in both children and birds.
Lead is one of the most common sources of toxicity seen in water birds and
raptors [28–30]; however, it may be seen in pet psittacines as well [4,9]. In pet
birds, sources of lead include stained glass, lead solder, curtain weights, and

fishing sinker weights. In older houses, Venetian blinds, linoleum, and paint may contain lead (Fig. 2A–D). During the writing of this article, toys sold at a bird fair, marketed as bird-safe toys, were responsible for the death of one sun conure and severe illness of another in the authors' practice (Fig. 3A–C). Lead solder was used to form the "feet" of the bathtub on this chain. Due to the sweet smell and taste of the lead solder and the malleability of lead, the birds ingested a significant amount of this material in the first 24 hours they had exposure to the toy. Severe hemoglobinuria, polyuria, polydypsia, depression, anorexia, and pronounced and rapidly progressive anemia were present in both birds. Seizures occurred before death in the conure that succumbed.

Toxicity is often associated with ingestion of lead shot or fishing weights in water birds [29–31], and carcasses contaminated with lead shot in raptors [28,30,32]. Clinical signs of lead poisoning are similar to those of zinc toxicosis; however, clinical signs are more severe and neurologic signs are more common with lead. In wild birds, population die-offs may occur [32,33]. One study demonstrated that even low levels of lead (<10 µg/dL) can cause damage to the central nervous system in chickens [18]. Teratogenesis and embryonic death have been noted in eggs from lead toxicity [34].

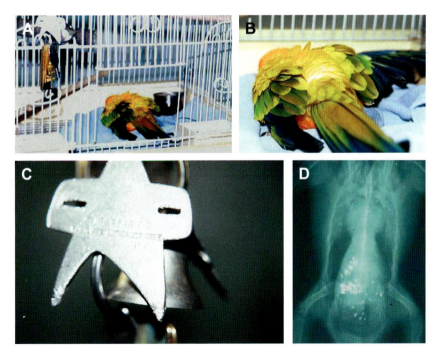

Fig. 2. (*A*) Conure presented in cage, found moribund. (*B*) Close up of conure in *A*. (*C*) Lead star that was purchased as a toy and attached to the conure's cage. (*D*) Ventrodorsal (VD) radiograph of conure demonstrating significant number of metal densities in GI tract.

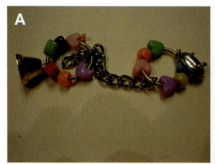
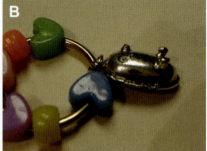
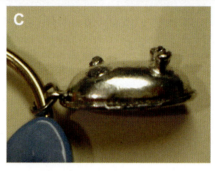

Fig. 3. (*A*) Toy sold at bird fair. (*B*) Closer view of same toy. (*C*) Close-up of miniature bathtub on toy. Note legs of tub have been chewed.

Hemaglobinuria, documented in *Amazona* sp, *Pionus* sp, *Aratinga* sp, *Eclectus* sp, and African Gray parrots (*Psitticus erithricus*) is another clinical sign that has been noted in psittacine birds [19]. Radiographic findings are similar to those noted with zinc toxicosis and blood work abnormalities may include anemia, heterophilia, and elevation of aspartate aminotransferase (AST), lactate dehydrogenase (LDH), creatine phosphokinase (CPK), and uric acid [4]. For determination of blood lead concentration, whole blood may be submitted in a similar fashion as described for zinc above. Nontoxic levels in whole blood are reported to be less than 0.02 ppm in Hispaniolan Amazon parrots (*Amazona ventralis*) [23], while more than 0.2 ppm is suspect and more than 0.5 ppm is diagnostic. Seven Florida sandhill cranes (*Grus canadensis pratensis*) and six greater sandhill cranes (*Grus canadensis tabida*) were diagnosed with lead poisoning from exposure to paint with a high concentration of lead. Blood lead levels ranged from 146 µg/dL (1.46 ppm) to 378 µg/dL (3.78 ppm) [35]. Lead concentrations may also be measured in tissues, most importantly the liver where concentrations above 6 ppm wet weight are diagnostic [9] and in bone when lead exposure has been chronic.

Chelation therapy (Table 1) is the principal means of treatment for lead and often for zinc toxicity. Chelating agents work by binding the heavy metal, forming a nontoxic chelate that is excreted [36].

Table 1
Chelation therapy

Agent	Dosage	Route	Indications	Notes
CaEDTA	25–40 mg/kg q 8–12 h	IM diluted	Pb, Zn, Hg	Most commonly used parenteral chelator for Pb and Zn
Penicillamine	40 mg/kg PO q 12 h	PO	Pb, Zn, Cu	May cause regurgitation
DMSA (meso-dimercaptosuccinic acid) SUCCIMER	10 mg/kg	PO	Pb, Hg, Cu (may be less effective for Zn)	Narrow margin of safety
Desferrioxamine	20–100 mg/kg q 24 h	SQ or IV	Iron storage disease	Poor GI absorption
Deferiprone	50 mg/kg q 24 h	PO	Iron storage disease	Oral, but only a partial chelator[a]
Deferasirox	unknown	PO	Iron storage disease	Recent FDA approval for children with thalassemia

Abbreviations: Cu, copper; FDA, Food and Drug Administration; GI, gastrointestinal; Hg, mercury; IM, intramuscular; IV, intravenous; Pb, lead; PO, by mouth; q, every; SQ, subcutaneous; ZN, zinc.

[a] *Data from* http://sickle.bwh.harvard.edu/chelators.html.

Ca EDTA is the chelator that has been the primary parenteral agent used for lead (and zinc) toxicity in humans and animals. One recommended dose in birds is 35 to 40 mg/kg intramuscularly (IM) or intravenously (IV) every 12 hours for 5 days and repeated as needed [5,37]. Another recommended avian dosage regime is the administration of 75 mg/kg/day total dose, divided, every 4 to 8 hours [36]. Fluid therapy should be included to prevent possible nephrotoxicity, although this has not been documented to occur in avian species [38]. Another form of EDTA, NaEDTA, is used for the treatment of hypercalcemia. NaEDTA is stocked routinely in hospitals and its trade name is similar to that of Ca EDTA. Inadvertent use of NaEDTA resulted in the death of several children in 2003-2004 due to hypocalcemia, tetany, and cardiac failure. One situation involved a naturopathic physician who administered a compounded form of EDTA. In 2006, the Centers for Disease Control and Prevention (CDC) recommended in its *Morbidity and Mortality Weekly Report* that "Hospital pharmacies should evaluate whether continued stocking of NaEDTA is necessary, given the established risk for hypocalcemia, the availability of less toxic alternatives, and an ongoing safety review by the Food and Drug Administration (FDA). Health care providers and pharmacists should ensure that NaEDTA is not administered to children during chelation therapy."

Meso-dimercaptosuccinic acid (DMSA) is another chelator that may be used. Treatment with meso-2,3-dimercaptosuccinic acid (succimer) is reported to be successful in decreasing lead plasma levels and resolving clinical signs in affected birds when administered at 30 mg/kg twice a day by mouth for 7 days with a single 50 mg/kg dose of Ca EDTA administered initially in severe neurologic cases [39]. One study compared the efficacy of CaEDTA and DMSA in experimentally induced lead toxicity in cockatiels. Both agents were efficacious. The oral route of administration for DMSA facilitated home treatment; however, DMSA has a narrow margin of safety [40]. Another retrospective study of 19 birds of various species treated with DMSA alone showed 87% decreased in serum lead concentration, and resolution of clinical signs, including neurologic abnormalities [39].

D-penicillamine is another chelator that can be administered for heavy metal toxicity at 55 mg/kg by mouth every 12 hours for 7 to 14 days. In children, it is used for low to moderate levels of lead toxicity, and although efficacious, is associated with a 33% rate of adverse reaction—most commonly GI upset, rash, transient leucopenia, and thrombocytopenia [41]. In birds, GI upset is commonly reported.

Human medical studies have also shown that, when chelation therapy is administered for lead toxicity, the concurrent administration of zinc is beneficial [42,43]. Chelation therapy often depletes the body's normal stores of zinc. The administration of zinc replaces these stores, and accelerates the chelation and excretion of lead [42,43].

Combination chelation therapy is being studied, and preliminary results are mixed as to the advantages or these regimes [44,45].

If large metal particles are identified within the GI tract, removal is important and is accomplished by gastric lavage, endoscopic removal, retrieval with long biopsy forceps or a magnet [25], or by surgical removal. If particles are too small to be retrieved, cathartics such as lactulose or psyllium [5] can be administered to accelerate excretion.

Other reported avian metal toxicities include cadmium [46–48], copper [5], mercury [49,50], and iron [51]. Except for iron, these rarely occur in pet birds and are often a result of environmental contamination [9,46,49,52] or food source concentration of the metal [53]. CaEDTA has been recommended for the treatment of cadmium toxicity [36]. Mercury is of increasing concern in wildlife that feeds from aquatic species such as bivalves and fish, which can accumulate mercury. Mercury toxicity may be treated with DMSA [9]. (Note: mercury found in glass thermometers is not absorbed by the GI tract, and is therefore nontoxic.) One study demonstrated that when chickens were poisoned with mercury, the administration of vitamin E and selenium had a sparing effect, decreasing the incidence of reproductive and developmental disorders [54]. Recent development of an aminosteroidal heterocyclic compound has shown promise in preventing the oxidative effects of iron toxicity in mammals [55]; however, its use has not been studied in avian species.

There is evidence than some pelagic birds may be able to form stable compounds in the liver that decrease circulating mercury [53].

Human food

Human foods can be a source of toxins for avian pets, as owners frequently share table food with their birds. Chocolate is a well-known food toxin that causes clinical signs in many other animals as well as birds. The toxic components of chocolate are theobromine and caffeine, both methylxanthines [56]. While there is no research to demonstrate how methylxanthines specifically affect birds, this class of compounds has been shown in mammals to be adenosine receptor antagonists [57]. Adenosine receptors are found throughout the body; however, receptors in nervous and cardiovascular tissue seem to be most affected by methylxanthines. Antagonism of these receptors in the cardiovascular system results in clinical signs such as tachycardia, hypertension [56,57], and ventricular arrhythmias [56]. Adenosine receptors in the central nervous system (CNS) have a locomotor depressant, anxiolytic, and sedative effect, thus inhibition results in CNS stimulation, hyperactivity, and anxiousness [56–58]. Seizures and hyperalgesia are also possible [57,58]. Renal adenosine receptor-inhibition results in decreased kidney function and polyuria has been noted [56,57]. Methylxanthines also inhibit benzodiazepine receptors and inhibit phosphodiesterase in the CNS [56,58]. Other reported effects in mammals include increased platelet aggregation [57], vomiting, diarrhea, muscle tremors, hyperthermia, increased respiratory rate, cyanosis, coma, and death [56]. Clinical signs may develop in minutes to hours and may be lethal within hours of ingestion [58].

Few cases of chocolate toxicosis have been reported in birds. However, chocolate toxicity is one of the most common poisonings reported in dogs presented to emergency clinics. This discrepancy may be due to a combination of factors. Birds may be less likely to ingest large amounts of chocolate. Also, birds' relative sensitivity to chocolate has not been documented. In the few reported cases of avian chocolate toxicosis, all resulted in death [59–61]. One patient demonstrated lethargy and mucoid feces before death [58,59], the others were found dead. Necropsy findings in one case included hepatic, renal, and pulmonary congestion [59]. Degeneration of hepatocytes, renal tubular cells, and cerebrocortical cells were found in another case [59]. In one psittacine case in which the patient was found dead, chocolate was present in the crop at necropsy and was determined to contain 250 mg/kg theobromine and 20 mg/kg of caffeine [59]. The LD50 dose of theobromine and caffeine in dogs are both reported to be 100 to 200 mg/kg. Clinical signs may be seen in canine patients at doses as low as 20 mg/kg [56]. Before initiating specific treatment, stabilization may be required. Seizures may be treated with diazepam at 0.5 mg/kg IV [37]. Dyspneic patients may be placed in oxygen [4]. Anxious or hyperactive patients may require sedation. Ventricular arrhythmias may be detected on ECG, however a paper speed of 100 to 200 mm/s is required for birds and normal values have not been established for most avian species [62]. Additionally, restraint and positioning for an ECG may cause excessive stress to a patient that is already compromised. In canine patients, ventricular arrhythmias are treated with beta-blockers such as metoprolol succinate or metoprolol tartrate. Propranolol HCl is not recommended because it slows renal clearance of methylxanthines. Parenteral fluid administration is recommended to diurese and clear the methylxanthines more quickly [4].

Treatment includes removal of any remaining chocolate from the GI tract. This is accomplished by crop and proventricular lavage, followed by administration of activated charcoal at 1 to 3 g/kg. Both of these procedures must be performed with care to prevent aspiration and generally require anesthesia and tracheal intubation [4,5,9]. Emesis should generally not be induced in avian patients because of the likelihood of resulting aspiration [5]. Activated charcoal is sometimes administered multiple times in canine patients because of enterohepatic recirculation [56].

Avocado

Pet birds may be exposed to toxins through ingestion of plants, some of which may be a normal part of human diets. Avocado (*Persea americana*) is known to be toxic to some avian species. All parts of the plant, including fruit, seeds, leaves, and bark can induce signs of toxicity [5]. Not all species of birds are equally affected by the toxins; thus, a single toxic dose cannot be established. Avocados of several species have been shown to be lethal within 24 to 48 hours in budgerigars that were fed 1.0-mL doses of an avocado and water mixture [63]. Larger parrots are more likely to demonstrate antemortem clinical signs such as lethargy, fluffed feathers, and increased respiratory effort [5]. The most consistent necropsy findings include pericardial effusion, subcutaneous, edema and generalized congestion of organs, including the lungs and liver.

P americana has been documented to cause sterile mastitis and agalactia in cattle that ingest it, and the source of this toxicity in cattle has been identified as a substance called persin, or (Z,Z)-1-(acetyloxy)-2-12,15-heneicosadien-4-one. This substance has also been shown to be toxic to mice and silk worms. At high doses (100 mg/kg) in mice it causes myocardial necrosis and pleural effusion [64,65]. Whether the same toxin is responsible for the toxic effects of avocados in birds has not been established.

Treatment of avian patients includes stabilization with oxygen, fluids, and other supportive care. Removal of the toxin from the GI tract is also important. This is accomplished by crop or proventricular lavage and administration of activated charcoal as described above.

Onion and garlic (*Allium* sp) are commonly consumed in human diets, to which pet birds may be exposed when owners share food with them. Garlic has also been used for human nutriceutical purposes ranging from parasite control [66] to antioxidant effects [67], which may lead owners to assume that it is beneficial for their pet birds as well. Any plant in the *Allium* genus is capable of causing toxicity. Some common North American plants in this genus include *Allium canadensis* (wild onion) and *Allium validum* (pacific onion) [68]. However, house birds are likely to be exposed to species more commonly consumed by humans such as *Allium cepa* (domesticated onion), *Allium porrum* (leek), *Allium schoenoprasum* (chive), and *Allium sativum* (garlic) [69]. All parts of the plant are toxic. Toxicity is due to sulfur-containing alkaloids such as alkenylcysteine sulfoxide [69], diallyl sulfinate [67], and N-propyl disulphide [66], among others. These compounds are activated by mechanical manipulation, cutting or crushing of the plant [67,69]. They are oxidizing agents that primarily affect hemoglobin molecules in most species reported to be susceptible [67–70]. In dogs, cats, cattle, and goats, hemolytic anemia results as the sulfur compounds oxidize hemoglobin and deform the molecule resulting in Heinz body formation [68,69]. Heinz body–containing erythrocytes become rigid, swell, and burst. They are also unable to pass through the microvasculature of the spleen and are phagocytised [67]. While Heinz body formation is possible in avian species, it is not a common finding in *Allium* toxicity [71]. In the few case reports of *Allium* sp ingestion toxicosis that have been published, birds developed anemia, anisocytosis, and an increased reticulocyte count; however, Heinz bodies were rarely seen [67]. There is not an established toxic dose in avian species; however, toxicity is seen in canine patients at 30 g/kg, and in cats at 5 g/kg [69].

Clinical signs of *Allium* toxicity observed in affected animals include lethargy, weakness, tachycardia, pale mucous membranes, collapse, and death [67,68,70]. Clinical pathology abnormalities are consistent with intravascular and extravascular hemolysis, including hemolytic anemia and occasional Heinz bodies [70]. Despite the infrequent detection of Heinz bodies in avian patients, necropsy findings in one case demonstrated that splenic erythrophagocytosis still occurs [67]. While icterus and increased total bilirubin are common findings in small mammals, avian species lack the enzyme biliverdin reductase to convert biliverdin to bilirubin, and thus icterus is not frequently seen [72]. Hemoglobin is also a nephrotoxin [67] and thus in addition to hemoglobinurea, hemoglobinuric nephrosis may be present in avian patients [69]. The liver may demonstrate erythrophagocytosis as well [67]. Hemosiderin deposition in the liver can also occur in chronically exposed animals [67,70]. Severe liver necrosis and centrolobular vacuolization were also present in White Chinese geese fed green onions for 3 weeks [70]. Other changes included pericardial effusion and petechiation of the epicardium [70].

Initial treatment of onion toxicity is similar to that of other ingested toxins, which includes initial stabilization and oxygen therapy followed by removal of any toxin still present in the GI tract via crop and proventricular lavage and activated charcoal administration. If anemia is severe, a blood transfusion may be indicated [67,69]. Administration of antioxidants such as vitamin E and ascorbic acid is recommended [67]; however, these antioxidants have not been shown to be beneficial in the treatment of cats with onion toxicity [69].

Salt toxicity is suspected in the case of a sun conure (*Aratinga solstitialis*) that presented to one author's practice. The bird was moribund after consuming a large number of salted mixed nuts. Notable laboratory serum values included Na of 184 mEq/L and a chloride of 135 mEq/L.

Toxic plants

Exposure to toxic plants may also occur when a curious bird ingests houseplants or landscaping (Table 2). There are few reports of pet bird plant toxicosis; however, these individuals are most likely to be exposed to plants in their immediate environment. Crown vetch (*Coronilla varia*) was found to be poisonous to a budgerigar that ingested leaves from a plant next to its cage [73]. This plant is known to be toxic in livestock that eat the plant while foraging [68]. Toxicity is due to nitroglycoside, a chemical that may affect the nervous system and can cause formation of methemoglobin [66,73]. Another group of plant neurotoxins that has been documented to affect other animal species is grayanotoxin, which may cause clinical signs such as seizures, ataxia, paralysis, or coma. Cardiac effects may also be noted [74]. Most grayanotoxin-containing plants are in the Ericaceae family, which include the commonly found *Rhododendron* [74].

Kalanchoe species have also been documented to cause toxicity in birds. There are many plants in this genus, several of which are toxic. They are commonly kept as houseplants for their colorful flowers and ease of care [75]. One study demonstrated that several species induced clinical signs in chickens that included ataxia, depression, muscle tremors, seizures, paralysis, and death [76]. Toxic doses were reported to be 8 to 12 mg/kg [76]. *Kalanchoe* species have been reported to contain bufadienolide cardiac glycosides [75,77]. Other plants that have been known to cause cardiac toxicities include *Nerium oleander* (oleander), *Taxus media* (yew), *Convallaria majalis* (lily of the valley), and *Digitalis purpurea* (foxgloves) [4,5,9], all of which are commonly used in landscaping, gardens, or flower arrangements. Cardiac signs may include increased contractility, bradycardia, wide QRS complexes, ventricular arrhythmias, and death [74,75,78].

While there are many plants that can cause hepatic toxicosis, pet birds are most likely to be exposed to hepatotoxic plants found around the home or aviary. Plants containing tannic acid have been documented to cause periacinar hepatic necrosis in chickens [79]. The acorns and leaves of oak trees (*Quercus* spp) are known to contain tannins (tannic acid and gallic acid; not to be confused with the tannins found in tea, which are generally beneficial flavonoid precursors) and have been shown to cause toxicity in avian as well as other species [80] when consumed [74,81]. Hepatic sinusoidal congestion, diffuse heptacellular swelling, and granularity and dissociation of hepatocytes were found in a double-waddled cassowary (*Casuarius casuarius*) that died after ingestion of oak leaves. In addition to the liver, the kidneys and gastrointestinal tract may be affected by oak leaf or acorn ingestion [79,81].

Table 2
Toxic plants

Plant	Toxin	Systems effected	Clinical signs
Coronilla varia (crown vetch)	Nitroglycoside	Nervous system, GI	Weakness, incoordination, ataxia, collapse
Ericaceae family: *Rhododendron, Pieris, Menziesia, Leucothoe, Ledum, Kalmia*	Grayanotoxins	Nervous system, cardiovascular, GI	Weakness, ataxia, paralysis, coma, bradycardia, hypotension, other cardiac abnormalities, mucosal irritation, ptyalism, emesis
Kalanchoe spp, *Nerium oleander* (oleander), *Taxus media* (yew), *Convallaria majalis* (lily of the valley), *Digitalis purpurea* (foxgloves), *Rhododendron*	Cardiac glycoside	Cardiovascular ± nervous system	Increased contractility, arrhythmias, cardiac arrest, tremors, ataxia, seizures, and coma have been reported in *Kalanchoe* toxicity in chickens
Quercus sp (oak trees)	Tannic acid and gallic acid	Liver, kidney, lungs, GI	Anorexia, polydypsia, diarrhea, weakness
Amanita muscaria (fly agaric mushroom)	Amanatin	Liver, kidney, GI	Vomiting, hematochezia, clinical signs associated with hypoglycemia, death
Lantana camara (Lantana)	Triterpene acids (lantadene A, lantadene B)	Liver	Necrosis of nonpigmented/unfeathered skin exposed to UV light
Lilium spp (Asiatic, Easter, tiger, and star-gazer lilies)	Unknown	Kidney	Signs of acute renal failure, toxicity only documented in domestic cats
Rheum spp (Rhubarb)	Oxalate crystals	Kidney, GI	Vomiting, swelling/edema of oral mucous membranes, clinical signs consistent with acute renal failure
Schefflera (umbrella plant), *Spathephyllum* (peace lily), *Dieffenbachia* (dumb cane), *Epiprenum* (pothos), *Philodendron* spp	Oxalate crystals	GI, serum calcium, kidney	Regurgitation, ptyalism, oral mucosa and choanal edema

This list of toxic plants represents plants that are commonly found in and around a home environment or have specifically been shown to be toxic to birds. There are many other plants considered to be toxic that are not listed here and this list should not be considered all inclusive.

Abbreviation: GI, gastrointestinal tract.

Amanita muscaria or the fly agaric mushroom [82] produces the well-known hepatotoxins, amantins. These toxins inhibit RNA polymerase and result in cell death. These mushrooms are found in almost every geographic region and primarily grow in association with birch, pine, spruce, fir, and larch trees [82]. Clinical signs are divided into four stages in people [83] and this course may be followed in other species, or ingestion may be rapidly fatal [84,85]. The initial stage is a latency period of 8 to 12 hours in most affected mammals. This is followed by severe gastrointestinal signs: vomiting, bloody diarrhea, and severe abdominal pain. Generally, a lag period follows that can vary from several hours to several days, depending on the dose and the individual's sensitivity, when the patient appears to have recovered. During this time the amantins are preferentially causing the greatest cell death in tissues with the highest metabolic rate: the hepatocytes and proximal tubules of the kidney. Massive hepatic glycogen breakdown may cause death due to hypoglycemia. This is followed by hepatic and renal failure, and necropsy findings may often demonstrate panlobular coagulative necrosis of hepatocytes [83]. Liver tissue samples may be tested for amanitin by mass spectrometry or liquid chromatography to confirm diagnosis [86].

Although a food source for some indigenous species, such as Gopher tortoises (*Gopherus polyphemus*), *Lantana camara* may cause hepatotoxicity in avian and other species [68,87,88]. This plant is found in tropical areas of North America and is commonly used in landscaping and grows wild in many southern US states [88]. Photosensitization and resulting necrosis of unfeathered skin was observed in a group of ostriches that consumed hay contaminated with lantana [87]. Photosensitization and hepatotoxicity are well-documented phenomena in livestock consuming lantana; however, not all species are toxic and a large amount must be consumed to induce toxicity in cattle. Hepatic damage caused by *Lantana* spp impairs the liver's ability to breakdown phylloerythrin, a chlorophyll by-product that is removed from circulation in a normally functioning liver. This compound is photoreactive and when high levels are present in circulation it is responsible for the observed necrosis of unpigmented skin exposed to UV light [68].

Kidneys may also be affected by toxic plants. Plants in the *Lilium* genus, such as the following lilies: Asiatic, Easter, tiger, and star-gazer, have been well-documented to cause acute renal failure in cats [89]. The toxic component(s), mechanism of toxicity, and pathogenesis have not been determined [89] and there are no reports of *Lilium* renal toxicosis in avian patients. As mentioned earlier, plants containing tannic acid may cause renal damage [79,81]. Rhubarb, a plant commonly grown in gardens may be nephrotoxic [5]. Toxicity is due to oxalate crystals, which are found in high concentrations in rhubarb leaves. Consumption of leaves may result in oxalate nephrosis [68]. Other plants containing high levels of oxalate crystals, such as beetroot and spinach may also result in renal failure [90]. However, renal toxicity varies with the species that ingests the oxalate-containing plant, the pH of the stomach, and the bacterial population of the GI tract, all of which may influence the solubility and absorption of oxalate [83,90,91].

Many plants responsible for other organ toxicities may cause GI signs as well. Oxalate crystal–containing plants are irritants to the GI tract [5]. Crystals cause pain, inflammation, and edema of the oropharyngeal mucosa on contact. Ptylism, dysphagia, and regurgitation may also be seen [4,74,77]. Soluble oxalate crystals may bind calcium and magnesium after absorption from the GI tract. Livestock that consume large quantities of oxalate-containing plants may develop hypocalcemia and hypomagnesaemia and die. Renal tubular damage may also occur [68]. Pet birds are unlikely to consume large volumes because of the pain associated with ingestion [74]. Common houseplants that contain oxalates include *Schefflera* (umbrella plant), *Spathephyllum* (peace lily), *Dieffenbachia* (dumb cane), *Epiprenum* (pothos), *Philodendron*, and others [4,9,68,74,77]. A commonly seen presentation is the ingestion of a small amount of pothos or philodendron houseplant. This has been noted most commonly by one author in cockatiels, which present with sudden onset of fluffing, pytalism, head shaking and "flinging" oral mucous. The tongue and choana are often erythematous. Symptomatic and supportive care has resulted in recovery in all cases to date, but more aggressive therapy may be warranted.

Other plants that have been shown to induce toxicity in birds and that may cause GI signs include *Robina pseudoacacia* (black locust), *Euphorbia pulcherima* (poinsettia), *Parthenocissus quinquefolio* (Virginia creeper), and *Montana rubens* (clematis) [9].

In any plant toxicity, after initial stabilization, removal of any remaining plant from the GI tract is indicated and is accomplished through crop and GI lavage. Activated charcoal is also effective in most plant intoxications, neutralizing toxic components remaining in the GI tract. Further treatment is directed at the organ systems affected and clinical signs.

Mycotoxins

Mycotoxins are toxins produced by fungi and commonly occur in fungal-contaminated grain products [9,92]. A commercial dog food with a high aflatoxin level was responsible for the acute deaths of 23 dogs in the United States in 2005. Avian species are more susceptible than other affected species, such as dogs, cattle, swine, and humans, to aflatoxicosis [93]. Aflatoxin and fusariotoxin are often responsible for avian mycotoxicosis and are usually associated with cereal grains, corn, and peanuts that have been exposed to or kept in humid, moist conditions [92]. *Aspergillus flavus* produces aflatoxins and *Fusarium* produces fusariotoxins [92,94]. Clinical signs of chronic aflalotoxicosis often include lethargy, weight loss, anorexia, regurgitation, and polydipsia [92,94]. The CNS may also be affected in some species [95] and signs such as ataxia may be noted [92]. Mycotoxins are hepatotoxic and histologic changes include increased content of hepatic glycogen, portal infiltrate of monocytes, increased lipid droplet accumulation, hepatic necrosis and bile duct hyperplasia [92,96]. Changes in levels of specific neurotransmitters in the pons and brain stem have also been noted in some species [95]. Testing for mycotoxins in food and in the patient can be difficult because of variation in toxic concentration and the inconsistent production of toxins [9].

While there is no specific treatment for mycotoxicosis, birds that are at high risk of exposure may benefit from supplementation with glucomannans and organic selenium, which appear to decrease the hepatotoxic and CNS changes associated with exposure [96,97]. While domestic animal feeds are required to contain less than 100 ppb of mycotoxins, hepatic changes have been shown to occur in turkeys at levels as low as 100 to 400 ppb [98]. In the United States, the acceptable level of total aflatoxins in food for human consumption is less than 20 µg/kg, except for Aflatoxin M1 in milk, which should be less than 0.5 µg/kg. The official document can be found at the Food and Drug Administration's (FDA) Web site: www.fda. gov. Other animal species have been documented to suffer from toxicity caused by various mycotoxins such as Penitrem A and roquefortine, both tremorgenic toxins, after consuming moldy human food [99]. The best way to protect pet birds from exposure to mycotoxins is to feed only human-grade grain, corn, and peanut products; avoid spoiled foods; and store grain products in cool, dry places.

Oil

Much is known and is still being studied regarding the adverse effect of crude oil on sea and coastal birds. Major oil spills over the past half-century have unfortunately given us a plethora of opportunities for research. Although the marine oil spills are the most notorious, the most oil contamination of the environment comes from land-based activity. The lighter fractions of oil, such as benzene and toluene, are more toxic, but are more volatile and evaporate quickly. Heavier components of crude oil, such as polynuclear aromatic hydrocarbons (PAHs), may cause the most extensive adverse effects; while they are less toxic, they persist in the environment much longer than volatile components. The initial effects on seabirds include damaging the feathers' ability to insult and to allow flight. Ingestion of oil via preening causes GI irritation, GI ulceration, and hemolytic anemia [100]. Dehydration and emaciation are commonly seen in birds that are victims of oil spills. Recent research has demonstrated that long-term effects include greatly decreased acetylcholinesterase brain activity in some species [101].

While exposure to oil is more common in free-ranging birds, pet birds may be exposed under various circumstances. Exposure to cooking oil is usually the result of a pet bird flying into a cooking pan on the stove or left out in the kitchen. They may also be intoxicated through exposure to petroleum-based products [9]. While hot oil can result in severe burns (a common pet bird emergency presentation), the oil itself inhibits feather function and is ingested as the bird preens [9,100,102]. Ingestion of oil products may have several systemic effects. Diarrhea and dehydration are the most frequently noted clinical signs [9]. Ingestion of crude oil by marine birds has been reported to cause GI hemorrhage and liver and kidney dysfunction [100]. Crude oil has also been shown to cause hemolytic anemia in several avian species [102]. Oil ingestion may also result in immunosuppression and secondary fungal and bacterial infections [103]. Pneumonia is also seen when oil is aspirated [9]. Treatment includes removal of oil from feathers using a dilute dishwashing detergent and hot water (106°F) [102]. This may need to be repeated several times. Washing should not be attempted until the bird is stable. Recently, dry-cleaning techniques with the use of iron powder and magnetic removal have been studied for their value as a less stressful and more effective method of oil decontamination [104]; however, one must take into consideration the potential risk of toxicity from oral exposure to iron. Further treatment includes supportive care based on clinical signs including oxygen therapy, fluid therapy, antibiotic therapy, antifungal therapy, liver protectants, pain management, and nutritional support.

Pesticides

Pesticides are commonly encountered in the free-ranging avian patient; however, pet birds may be exposed to pesticides used in a home setting. The most common types of pesticides include organophosphates, carbamates, and pyrethrins [9,105]. Exposure may occur by inhalation or ingestion [9]. Organophosphates and carbamates are anticholinesterases and work by inhibiting cholinesterase [106]. Without cholinesterase to bind acetylcholine at the neuromuscular junctions, excessive acetylcholine leads to paralysis, which can eventually involve the muscles of respiration [107]. Clinical signs include weakness, lethargy, ataxia, tremors, seizures, and death [107]. Pupillary miosis, which is often noted in mammals with anticholinesterase toxicity, will not be seen in birds because of the striated muscle of the iris. Diarrhea and ptyalism have also been reported in association with exposure to organophosphates and carbamates in avian patients [108,109]. Thriam and other multiple sulfide group–containing carbamate pesticides have been shown to cause tibial dyschondroplasia and lower body weight in young growing broiler chickens and turkeys fed at high doses of 50 mg/kg and 400 mg/kg, respectively [110,111]. Reproductive effects have also been noted [107]. Diagnosis is made by history of exposure, identification of consistent clinical signs, and demonstration of reduced cholinesterase levels in brain tissue or serum [107,110].

Treatment consists of the administration of anticholinergics such as atropine, with suggested doses ranging from 0.01 to 0.1 mg/kg subcutaneously (SQ), IM, or IV [37,108,112]. However, in mammals, organ-ophosphate-induced signs usually do not respond to the lower end of the dose range [9,112]. Pralidoxime chloride (2PAM) is used as an antidote for organophosphate toxicity in dogs and cats, but is not recommended for treatment of carbamate toxicity [112].

Pyretherins work by gate alteration of sodium, calcium, and chloride channels [113]. Clinical signs of pyretherin toxicity in mammals include behavior change, tremors, hyperthermia, and seizures [112,113]. Pyretherins may also impair the immune system and alter numerous metabolic pathways in birds [114]. Pyrethrin toxicity often occurs in cats when high concentra-tion (45% to 50%) canine spot-on pyrethrins are applied [112]. Diagnosis is made by recognition of clinical signs and history of exposure. Diazepam may be administered for treatment of seizures; however, it has been shown to be only partially effective in pyretherin toxicity [112,113]. Methocarbamol has been used in mammals to control tremors. If topical exposure has oc-curred, once a bird is stable, bathing in dilute dish soap is indicated to re-move any residual toxin [112].

Wild bird toxicity still occurs from the metabolites of banned pesticides, such as DDT. In 1999, Lake Apopka, Florida, was the site of a major die-off of white pelicans (*Pelecanus erythrorhynchos*), wood storks (*Mycteria amer-icana*), great blue herons (*Ardea herodias*), and great egrets (*Casmerodius albus*). This was caused by flooding of farmland to provide replacement wet lands for the areas lost to extensive development. Unfortunately, although spot testing of the soil was performed, a high concentration of organochlorines, especially toxaphene, were released into the water of the newly formed wet lands, having been exuded from the underlying soil. Over 800 birds are known to have died in this incident, and the effect on propagation is still not known because of the migratory nature of several species, including the white pelican. Potential delayed effects of these organochlorines (OC) may include; thin-shelled eggs, decreased sperm pro-duction, cessation of egg laying, and decreased hatching rate. The reproduc-tive effects of OCs seem to be more pronounced in avian species than in mammals. Another potential sequelae to OC toxicity is osteodystrophy, which can be manifested by pathology in numerous bones. Carcinogenesis has been widely theorized but not proven [115].

Rodenticides

Pet birds may also be exposed to rodenticides in the home environment; however, most cases of rodenticide poisoning in birds occur in wild raptors and other birds that are nontarget species [116]. Anticoagulent rodenticides work by inhibition of the extrinsic, vitamin K–dependant pathway, in partic-ular factor VII. Because birds rely more on the intrinsic pathway, factor VII may play a less important role in avian species and thus explain their appar-ent decreased sensitivity to anticoagulant rodenticides [117]. However, cases of toxicity have been documented in raptors and other free-ranging birds. Sensitivity to rodenticide appears to vary among avian species, with documented brodifacoum (second-generation rodenticide) toxicity occurring at doses less than 1 mg/kg in some species and greater than 20 mg/kg in other species [116]. Clinical signs are similar to those seen in other animals and include hemorrhage, hematochezia, bruising, petechiation, and death [9,116]. While tests to assess function of clotting factors V, VII, and X have been developed in chickens, they are species-specific and have not been tested in other avian species [118]; thus, clotting factor function cannot be routinely evaluated in avian patients at this time.

Treatment is similar to that in mammals and consists of vitamin K supplementation. Treatment should be continued for 14 to 28 days [37].

Hypercalcemic rodenticides have been reported to cause death in birds [119]. These rodenticides are calciferol derivatives and produce hypercalcemia. The hypercalcemia leads to increased ionized calcium levels, metastatic calcification, cardiac conduction disturbances, renal failure, and death. Some rodenticides are a combination of anticoagulant and calciferol, with these two agents producing a synergistic effect.

Clinical signs of exposure to hypercalcemic rodenticides vary widely. Therefore, in addition to a markedly elevated serum calcium, a history of potential exposure is needed for diagnosis, and other causes of hypercalcemia must be ruled out (including paraneoplastic disease, lymphoma, hyperparathyroidism and, in birds, estrogen-related normal reproductive hypercalcemia).

Treatment of rodenticide hypercalcemia includes intense diuresis, glucocorticoids, and an antihypercalcemic. Pamidronate, a bisphosphonate, acts to inhibit bone resorbtion. This drug was designed for the hypercalcemia of malignancy in humans, and is preferred over calcitonin for treatment of rodenticide hypercalcemia.

Zinc phosphide is commonly used as a rodenticide on golf courses, highways, and other large areas where rodent control is required. It may be formulated as a grain-based bait or as a paste. Symptoms of acute zinc phosphide poisoning may include vomiting, diarrhea, cyanosis, low blood pressure, and loss of consciousness [120]. Zinc phosphide releases phosphine gas in the acid environment of the stomach. This gas is responsible for the toxic effects. Zinc phosphide has a strong, pungent odor that does not deter rodents, but which is offensive to many mammals. However, birds, notably wild turkeys, are not deterred by the odor. Of the avian species studied, the most sensitive to zinc phosphide toxicity are geese, pheasants, morning doves, quail, and mallard ducks [120].

There is no specific antidote for zinc phosphide toxicity. Supportive care includes gastric lavage to remove as much of the material as possible, followed by sodium bicarbonate to decrease the release of any addition phosphine gas. Calcium gluconate and sodium lactate may be administered IV to counteract systemic acidosis.

At the time of this writing, bromethalin is the most commonly sold over-the-counter rat and mouse bait. Bromethalin is a rodenticide that causes cerebral edema. Paralysis, seizures, and death ensue in the target species within 24 to 36 hrs. There is no specific test for this agent, nor is there an antidote; therefore, the primary treatment is the rapid induction of emesis. Although there is a risk of aspiration when emesis is induced in birds, if gastric lavage cannot be accomplished promptly and thoroughly, inducing emesis may be considered. Additional treatment involves the administration of activated charcoal and supportive care.

Although the LD_{50} in birds is not known, extrapolating from the dog (4.7 mg/kg) and cat (1.8 mg/kg) will assist the practitioner is assessing the degree of avian exposure to bromethalin [117].

Ethylene glycol

While uncommon, there have been reports of and research done that demonstrate avian susceptibility to renal failure induced by ethylene glycol ingestion [121]. Clinical signs include lethargy, ataxia, incoordination, and death [122]. Clinical pathology may demonstrate a metabolic acidosis and in mammals low blood calcium may be seen due to the formation of calcium oxalate crystals. Histopathologic findings include hepatocyte and renal tubular necrosis and degeneration with calcium oxalate crystals visualized in the tubules. Grossly, the kidneys and liver may be congested and enlarged [121]. Treatment in mammals includes fluid diuresis and the administration of ethanol or fomipizol. Prognosis varies depending on the amount ingested and the time elapsed from ingestion to treatment.

Iatrogenic toxicities

Any drug, medication, or supplement can be toxic at high enough doses. Avian patients may be more likely to suffer from iatrogenic toxicities because of their small size and resulting dosing mistakes. Many drugs that are commonly used in other species are not approved or studied in avian species and thus therapeutic and toxic doses are unknown. Recently, a study demonstrated that passerines and Columbiformes are sensitive to fenbendazole and albendazole [123]. Anecdotal reports of toxicity in cockatiels following repeated fenbendazole administration have been frequently reported [124]. A group of kiwi demonstrated acute respiratory distress and death after administration of levamisole at recommended doses of 25 to 43 mg/kg [125]. Furthermore, medications in aviary situations may be administered in food or water, which does not allow control over individual dosages.

Consumption of owners' medications by pet birds may be encountered. Birds that are prone to chew, because of age, species, or individual temperament, are more likely to be affected. The amount of a substance ingested is often difficult to determine. Knowledge of the clinical signs of overdose for a given drug in other species can be extrapolated to birds. The bird should be observed for the occurrence of any clinical signs that warrant treatment.

Vitamins and minerals

Toxicity may occur from over supplementation of vitamins and minerals. Fat-soluble vitamins, such as vitamin A and D, are more likely to cause toxicity when overdosed. Supplementation with these should be avoided when a balanced, pelleted diet is fed [126].

Vitamin D

Necropsy findings in chronic excessive vitamin D3 ingestion include soft tissue calcification and renal failure, and chronic vitamin D excess may contribute to atherosclerosis in mammals and birds [77,127,128]. Cholecalciferol should be used when oral vitamin D3 supplementation is necessary. Since cholecalciferol must be metabolized via the liver and kidney before activation, toxicity is unlikely. Vitamin D3 toxicity has been induced in macaws at lower dietary levels than in other species (1000I U/kg). This suggests that vitamin D3 metabolism varies among psittacine species. Poultry fed excessive vitamin D3 use the egg as an excretion vehicle, leading to embryonic death; a mechanism not available to most pet bird species. Pending further research, it seems prudent to feed parrots a formulated diet containing vitamin D3 at concentrations at or slightly below the poultry requirements. In addition to the provision of adequate dietary calcium and UVB light, this should to prevent metabolic bone disease and potential vitamin D3 toxicity problems.

Vitamin A

Although vitamin A deficiency is a common problem in pet birds, and studies to determine minimum requirements for health and breeding are ongoing [77,129], vitamin A toxicosis has been reported to cause both reproductive disease, osteodystrophy, and other behavioral and metabolic abnormalities in several species of birds [130].

In addition to altering the diet to decrease vitamin A content, administration of vitamin E has been shown to decrease serum vitamin A levels in rabbits [131]. When needed, supplementation of vitamin A should be in the form of beta-carotene, which is less likely to cause toxicity [77]. The vitamin A content of hand-rearing formulas, nectars, and pellets, should be evaluated. No recommendation can yet be made as to minimum or maximum dietary levels of vitamin A, but cockatiels fed 10,000 IU/kg as adults developed clinical signs of vitamin A toxicity. Many commercial products exceed this level [5].

Mineral toxicity is also possible with supplementation and potentially toxic minerals include selenium [132,133].

Iron

Soft-billed birds, such as the *Rhamphastos* (toucan) family, *Fracula religiosa* (Indian Hill Mynas), hornbills, starlings, and birds of paradise have been shown to be very sensitive to dietary levels of iron and commonly develop iron toxicosis [77,134–138]. In mynah birds, it has been demonstrated that excessive iron absorption from the GI tract is at least in part accountable for the prevalence of iron storage disease in captivity. When compared with chickens, mynah bird enterocytes have a significantly higher limiting uptake rate for iron, possibly because of an increased number of transporters [139]. In toucans, it has been demonstrated that lower-iron diets can successfully decrease hepatic iron content [140]. Although the exact mechanisms by which each susceptible avian species develops iron storage disease is not known, increased iron absorption and captive diets with higher iron content than is found in their natural diets, are likely factors. In some species, the wild diets may contain high levels of tannin-containing plant material, which inhibits iron absorption [134]. Tannins (not the same as tannic acid that occurs in other plants) are the precursors of flavonoids or catechins, which have been reported to possess divalent metal chelating, antioxidant, and anti-inflammatory activities; to penetrate the brain barrier; and to protect neuronal death in a wide array of cellular and animal models of neurologic diseases [141]. Current recommendations for diets of susceptible species should have maximum iron levels of 20 to 40 ppm [136].

Lories (Family Loriinae) have also been documented to have a disproportionate incidence of iron storage disease, although it is unclear whether this is due to unusually high dietary iron, other nutritional factors such as excess dietary vitamin C or A, or a species predilection [77,142,143].

Clinical signs of iron toxicosis/iron storage disease may include poor plumage, anorexia, lethargy, weight loss, ascites, dyspnea, and death. Elevated liver enzymes and/or elevated bile acids may be noted [136]. In clinically affected birds, an elevated PCV has been reported, but a causal relationship has not been documented (B. Speer, personal communication, November 2007). Serum iron levels may not be diagnostic and liver biopsy has the highest diagnostic yield [136]. Pathologic changes include accumulation of iron in the liver and iron deposition may also be noted in splenic, pancreatic, pulmonary, and renal tissues [136]. A precursor of iron storage disease is hemosiderosis, defined as the presence of excessive iron in the liver without alteration of tissue morphology. Iron storage disease, often referred to as hemochromatosis, is histologically distinguishable from hemosiderosis and involves hepatocellular damage. The term hemochromatosis has become synonymous with hereditary iron overload syndrome in people. Although the exact mechanism in people by which excessive iron is accumulated is unknown, human hemochromatosis is one of the most prevalent heritable genetic diseases and is caused by one of several gene mutations. To avoid confusion with the syndrome in people, in which the cause is known to be genetic and associated organ involvement may differ from that seen in birds, the term iron storage disease is currently preferred in avian medicine.

Treatment consists of repeated phlebotomies, use of iron chelators such as deferiprone or deferoxamine mesilate (see Fig. 1) [136], restricting vitamin A and C intake and a low-iron diet [77].

Summary

Birds may be exposed to toxins through a variety of sources in their every-day environment. Toxicity may occur through inhalation or oral or dermal exposures. It is the clinician's responsibility to diagnose and treat these toxicities to the best of his or her ability in an effort to correct the disease of the individual patient. Recognition of toxicity in the avian patient has further significance as it relates to the patient's environment, including the health of other animals, humans, and the ecosystem. Veterinarians diagnosing poisoning in animals have a responsibility to consider human health implications as well as treating their patient(s). While some toxicities, such as lead and zinc toxicosis, are well documented in avian species, others are limited to anecdotal reports and extrapolation from other species. Continued research is needed in this area of avian medicine to expand our knowledge and improve our ability to diagnose and treat toxic conditions in birds.

References

[1] Ehrsam H. Intoxications with lethal outcomes in small pet birds after accidental overheating of cooking pans coated with polytetrafluoroethylene coating. Schweizer Archiv fur Tierheilkunde 1969;111:181–6.

[2] Forbes NA, Jones D. PTFE toxicity in birds. Vet Rec 1997;140(19):512.

[3] Wells RE, Slocombe RF. Acute toxicosis of budgerigars (*Melopsittacus undulates*) caused by pyrolysis products from heated polytetrafluoroethylene: microsopic study. Am J Vet Res 1982;43(7):1243–8.

[4] Dumonceaux G, Harrison GJ. Toxins. In: Ritchie BW, Harrison GJ, Harrison LR, editors. Avian medicine principles and application. Delray Beach (FL): HBD International, Inc; 1999. p. 1030–49.

[5] Richardson J. Implications of toxic substances in clinical disorders. In: Harrison GJ, Lightfoot T, editors. Clinical avian medicine. Palm Beach (FL): Spix Publishing; 2006. p. 711–9.

[6] Blandford TB, Hughes R, Seamon PJ, et al. Case of polytetrafluoroethylene poisoning in cockatiels accompanied by polymer fume fever in the owner. Vet Rec 1975;96:175–6.

[7] Silver MJ, Young DK. Acute noncardiogenic pulmonary edema due to polymer fume fever. Cleve Clin J Med 1993;60(6):479–82.

[8] Townsend PW, Vernice GG, Williams RL. 'Polymer fume fever' without polymer. J Fluor Chem 1989;42(3):441–3.

[9] LaBonde J. Toxicity in pet avian patients. Seminars in Avian and Exotic Pet Medicine 1995; 4(1):23–31.

[10] Verstappen FALM, Dorrestein GM. Aspergillosis in Amazon parrots after corticosteroid therapy for smoke-inhalation injury. J Avian Med Surg 2005;19(2):138–41.

[11] Jones MP. Avian toxicology (V489). Western Veterinary Conference. Las Vegas, NV; February 11-15, 2007.

[12] Cray C, Roskos J, Zielezienski-Roberts K. Detection of cotinine, a nicotine metabolite, in the plasma of birds exposed to secondhand smoke. J Avian Med Surg 2005;19(4): 277–9.

[13] Penn A, Snyder CA. 1,3 Butadiene, a vapor phase component of environmental tobacco smoke, accelerates arteriosclerotic plaque development. Circulation 1996;93:552–7.

[14] Izrael M, Van der Zee E, Slotkin TA, et al. Cholinergic synaptic signaling mechanisms underlying behavioral teratogenicity: effects of nicotine, chlorpyrifos, and heroin converge on protein kinase C translocation in the intermedial part of the hyperstriatum ventral and on imprinting behavior in an avian model. J Neurosci Res 2004;78(4):499–507.

[15] Richardson JA, Murphy LA, Khan SA, et al. Managing pet bird toxicosis. Exotic DVM Veterinary Magazine 2001;3(1):23–7.

[16] Wilson H, Brown CA, Greenacre CB, et al. Suspected sodium hypochlorite toxicosis in a group of psittacine birds. J Avian Med Surg 2001;15(3):209–15.

[17] Aranyi C, O'Shea WJ, Graham JA, et al. The effects of inhalation of organic chemical air contaminant on murine lung host defenses. Fundam Appl Toxicol 1986;6:713–20.

[18] Lurie D, Brooks DM, Gray LC. The effect of lead on the avian auditory brainstem. Neurotoxicology 2006;27(1):108–17.

[19] Lightfoot T. Avian common clinical presentations: neoplastic, toxic, viral and miscellaneous. Atlantic Coast Veterinary Conference; Atlantic City, NJ; 2001.

[20] Morris D. Lead and zinc toxicosis in a blue and gold macaw (Ara ararauna) caused by ingestion of hardware cloth. Association of Avian Veterinarians Newsletter 1985;6(3):75.

[21] Holz P, Phelan J, Slocombe R, et al. Suspected zinc toxicosis as a cause of sudden death in orange-bellied parrots (Neophema chrysogaster). J Avian Med Surg 2000;14(1):37–41.

[22] Rosenthal KL, Johnston MS, Shofer FS, et al. Psittacine plasma concentrations of elements: daily fluctuations and clinical implications. J Vet Diagn Invest 2005;17(3):239–44.

[23] Osofsky A, Jowett P, Hosgood G, et al. Determination of normal blood concentrations of lead, zinc, copper, and iron in Hispaniolan Amazon (Amazona vetralis). J Avian Med Surg 2001;15(1):31–6.

[24] Frank EL, Hughes MP, Bankson DD, et al. Effects of anticoagulants and contemporary blood collection containers on aluminum, copper, and zinc results. Clin Chem 2001;47: 1109–12.

[25] Samour J, Naldo JL. Lead toxicosis in falcons: a method for lead retrieval. Seminars in Avian and Exotic Pet Medicine 2005;14(2):143–8.

[26] Carpenter JW. Zinc toxicosis in a free-flying trumpeter swan (Cygnus buccinators). J Wildl Dis 2004;40(4):769–74.

[27] Droual R, Meteyer CU, Galey FD. Zinc toxicosis due to ingestion of a penny in a gray-headed chachalaca (Ortalis cinereiceps). Avian Dis 1991;35(4):1007–11.

[28] Church ME, Gwiazda R, Risebrough RW, et al. Ammunition is the principal source of lead accumulated by California condors re-introduced to the wild. Environ Sci Technol 2006; 40(19):6143–50.

[29] Svanberg F, Mateo R, Hillström L, et al. Lead isotopes and lead shot ingestion in the globally threatened marbled teal (Marmaronetta angustirostris) and white-headed duck (Oxyura leucocephala). Sci Total Environ 2006;370(2–3):416–24.

[30] Cousquer GO. Severe lead poisoning and an abdominal foreign body in a mute swan (Cygnus olor). Vet Clin North Am Exot Anim Pract 2006;9(3):503–10.

[31] Murase T, Ikeda T, Goto I, et al. Treatment of lead poisoning in wild geese. J Am Vet Med Assoc 1992;200(11):1726–9.

[32] De Francisco N, Ruiz Troya JD, Agüera EI. Lead and lead toxicity in domestic and free living birds. Avian Pathol 2003;32(1):3–13.

[33] Spears BL, Hansen JA, Audet DJ. Blood lead concentrations in waterfowl utilizing Lake Coeur d'Alene, Idaho. Arch Environ Contam Toxicol 2007;52(1):121–8.

[34] Kertész V, Bakonyi G, Farkas B. Water pollution by Cu and Pb can adversely affect mallard embryonic development. Ecotoxicol Environ Saf 2006;65(1):67–73.

[35] Kennedy S, Crisler JP, Smith E, et al. Lead poisoning in sandhill cranes. J Am Vet Med Assoc 1977;171(9):955–8.

[36] El Bahri L. Edetate calcium disodium. Compend Contin Educ Pract Vet 2005;27(8):612–4.

[37] Carpenter JW. Exotic animal formulary. 3rd edition. St. Louis (MO): Elsevier; 2005. p. 202, 227, 229.

[38] McDonald SE. Lead poisoning in psittacine birds. In: Kirk RB, editor. Current veterinary therapy small animal practice IX. Philadelphia: WB Saunders Company; 1986. p. 713–8.

[39] Hoogesteijn AL, Raphael BL, Calle P, et al. Oral treatment of avian lead intoxication with meso-2,3-dimercaptosuccinic acid. J Zoo Wildl Med 2003;34(1):82–7.

[40] Denver MC, Tell LA, Galey FD, et al. Comparison of two heavy metal chelators for treatment of lead toxicosis in cockatiels. Am J Vet Res 2000;61(8):935–40.

[41] Shannon M, Graef J, Lovejoy FH. Efficacy and toxicity of D-penicillamine in low-level lead poisoning. J Pediatr 1988;112(5):799–804.

[42] Blanusa M, Varnai VM, Piasek M, et al. Chelators as antidotes of metal toxicity: therapeutic and experimental aspects. Curr Med Chem 2005;12(23):2771–94.

[43] Flora SJ, Tandon SK. Beneficial effects of zinc supplementation during chelation treatment of lead intoxication in rats. Toxicology 1990;64(2):129–39.

[44] Kalia K, Flora SJ. Strategies for safe and effective therapeutic measures for chronic arsenic and lead poisoning. J Occup Health 2005;47(1):1–21.

[45] Flora SJ, Saxena G, Mehta A. Reversal of lead-induced neuronal apoptosis by chelation treatment in rats: role of reactive oxygen species and intracellular Ca(2+). J Pharmacol Exp Ther 2007;322(1):108–16.

[46] Berzina N, Markovs J, Isajevs S, et al. Cadmium-induced enteropathy in domestic cocks: a biochemical and histological study after subchronic exposure. Basic Clin Pharmacol Toxicol 2007;101(1):29–34.

[47] Blechinger SR, Kusch RC, Haugo K, et al. Brief embryonic cadmium exposure induces a stress response and cell death in the developing olfactory system followed by long-term olfactory deficits in juvenile zebrafish. Toxicol Appl Pharmacol 2007; 224(1):72–80.

[48] Thompson JM, Bannigan JG. Omphalocele induction in the chick embryo by administration of cadmium. J Pediatr Surg 2007;42(10):1703–9.

[49] Scheuhammer AM, Meyer MW, Sandheinrich MB, et al. Effects of environmental methylmercury on the health of wild birds, mammals, and fish. Ambio 2007;36(1):12–8.

[50] Heath JA, Frederick PC. Relationships among mercury concentrations, hormones, and nesting effort of White Ibises (Eudocimus albus) in the Florida Everglades. Auk 2005; 122(1):255–67.

[51] Crissey SD, Ward AM, Block SE, et al. Hepatic iron accumulation over time in European starlings (Sturnus vulgaris) fed two levels of iron. J Zoo Widl Med 2000;31(4):491–6.

[52] Artacho P, Soto-Gamboa M, Verdugo C, et al. Blood biochemistry reveals malnutrition in black-necked swans (Cygnus melanocoryphus) living in a conservation priority area. Comp Biochem Physiol A Mol Integr Physiol 2007;146(2):283–90.

[53] Ikemoto T, Kunito T, Tanaka H, et al. Detoxification mechanism of heavy metals in marine mammals and seabirds: interaction of selenium with mercury, silver, copper, zinc, and cadmium in liver. Arch Environ Contam Toxicol 2004;47(3):402–13.

[54] Beyrouty P, Chan HM. Co-consumption of selenium and vitamin E altered the reproductive and developmental toxicity of methylmercury in rats. Neurotoxicol Teratol 2006;28(1): 49–58.

[55] Elmegeed GA, Ahmed HH, Hussein JS. Novel synthesized aminosteroidal heterocycles intervention for inhibiting iron-induced oxidative stress. Eur J Med Chem 2005;40(12): 1283–94.

[56] Gwaltney-Brant S. Chocolate intoxication. Vet Med 2001;96:108–11.

[57] Yaar R, Jones MR, Chen JF, et al. Animal models for the study of adenosine receptor function. J Cell Physiol 2005;202:9–20.

[58] Beasley V. Toxicants associated with stimulation or seizures. In: Beasley V, editor. Veterinary toxicology. Ithaca (NY): International Veterinary Information Services; 1999. Chapter 5.

[59] Gartrell BD, Reid C. Death by chocolate: a fatal problem for an inquisitive wild parrot. N Z Vet J 2007;55(3):149–51.

[60] Cole G, Murray M. Suspected chocolate toxicosis in an African Grey parrot (*Psittacus erithacus*) (700). Association of Avian Veterinarians Conference and Expo. Monterey, CA; August 8-12, 2005.

[61] Pybus MJ, Hanson JA, Rippin B. The case of the killer cookies: apparent chocolate poisoning of gulls. Canadian Cooperative Wildlife Health Centre Newsletter 1995;3(3):6.

[62] Oglesbee B. Overview of avian cardiology. Western Veterinary Conference. Las Vegas, NV; February 9-14, 2003.

[63] Hargis AM, Stauber E, Casteel S, et al. Avocado (*Persea americana*) intoxication in caged birds. J Am Vet Med Assoc 1989;194:64–6.

[64] Oelrichs PB, Ng JC, Seawright AA, et al. Isolation and identification of a compound from avocado (*Persea americana*) leaves which causes necrosis of the acinar epithelium of the lactating mammary gland and the myocardium. Nat Toxins 1995;3(5):344–9.

[65] Grant R, Basson PA, Booker HH, et al. Cardiomyopathy caused by avocado (*Persea americana* Mill) leaves. J S Afr Vet Assoc 1991;62(1):21–2.

[66] Nchu F, Magano SR, Eloff JN. In vitro investigation of the toxic effects of extracts of *Allium sativum* bulbs on adults of *Hyalomma marginatum rufipes* and *Rhipicephalus pulchellus*. J S Afr Vet Assoc 2005;76(2):99–103.

[67] Wade LL, Newman SJ. Hemoglobinuric nephrosis and hepatosplenic erythrophagocytosis in a dusky-headed conure (*Aratinga weddelli*) after ingestion of garlic (*Allium sativum*). J Avian Med Surg 2004;18(3):155–61.

[68] Knight AP, Walter RG. A guide to plant poisoning of animals in North America. Jackson (WY): Teton NewMedia; 2001. p. 142–85, 187–202, 203–17, 263–77.

[69] Cope RB. *Allium* species poisoning in dogs and cats. Vet Med 2005;100:562–6.

[70] Crespo R, Chin RP. Effect of feeding green onions (*Allium ascalonicum*) to White Chinese geese (*Threskiornis spinicollis*). J Vet Diagn Invest 2004;16:321–5.

[71] Campbell TW, Ellis C. Hematology of birds. In: Campbell TW, Ellis C, editors. Avian and exotic hematology and cytology. 3rd edition. Ames (IA): Blackwell Synergy; 2007. p. 14–6.

[72] Duke GE. Alimentary canal: secretion and digestion, special digestive functions, and absorption. In: Sturkie PD, editor. Avian physiology. New York: Springer-Verlag; 1986. p. 289–302.

[73] Campbell TW. Crown vetch (*Coronilla varia*) poisoning in a budgerigar (*Melopsittacus undulatus*). J Avian Med Surg 2006;20(2):97–100.

[74] Poppenga RH. Toxic household, garden, and ornamnetal plants. Western Veterinary Conference. Las Vegas, NV; February 10-14, 2002.

[75] Smith G. *Kalanchoe* species poisoning in pets. Vet Med 2004;99(11):933–6.

[76] Williams MC, Smith MC. Toxicity of *Kalanchoe* spp to chicks. Am J Vet Res 1984;45(3): 543–6.

[77] MacDonald D. Nutritional considerations. In: Harrison GJ, Lightfoot T, editors. Clinical avian medicine. Palm Beach (FL): Spix Publishing; 2006. p. 86–139.

[78] Ruch SR, Nishio M, Wasserstrom JA. Effect of cardiac glycosides on action potential characteristics and contractility in cat ventricular myocytes: role of calcium overload. J Pharmacol Exp Ther 2003;307(1):419–28.

[79] Philbey AW, Andrew PL, Gestier AW, et al. Spironucleosis in Australian king parrots (*Alisterus scapularis*). Aust Vet J 2002;80(3):154–60.

[80] Hervás G, Pérez V, Giráldez FJ, et al. Intoxication of sheep with quebracho tannin extract. J Comp Pathol 2003;129(1):44–54.
[81] Kinde H. A fatal case of oak poisoning in a double-wattled cassowary (*Casuarius casuarius*). Avian Dis 1988;32(4):849–51.
[82] Geml J, Laursen GA, O'Neill K, et al. Beringian origins and cryptic speciation events in the fly agaric (*Amanita muscaria*). Mol Ecol 2006;15:225–39.
[83] Puschner B. Mushroom toxins. In: Gupta RC, editor. Veterinary toxicology; basic and clinical principles. New York: Elsevier; 2007. p. 915–25.
[84] Tegzes J, Puschner B. *Amanita* mushroom poisoning: efficacy of aggressive treatment of two dogs. Vet Hum Toxicol 2002;44(2):96–9.
[85] Parish RC, Doering PL. Treatment of *Amanita* mushroom poisoning: a review. Vet Hum Toxicol 1986;28(4):318–22.
[86] Puschner B, Rose HH, Filigenzi MS. Diagnosis of *Amanita* toxicosis in a dog with acute hepatic necrosis. J Vet Diagn Invest 2007;19:312–7.
[87] Cooper RG. Accidental poisoning from *Lantana camara* (Cherry Pie) in hay fed to ostriches (*Struthio camelus*). Turkish Journal of Veterinary and Animal Sciences 2007;31(3):213–4.
[88] Sharma OP, Sharma S, Pattabhi V, et al. A review of the hepatotoxic plant *Lantana camara*. Crit Rev Toxicol 2007;37(4):313–52.
[89] Rumbeiha WK, Francis JA, Fitzgerald SD, et al. A comprehensive study of Easter lily poisoning it cats. J Vet Diagn Invest 2004;16:527–41.
[90] Holowaychuk MK. Renal failure in a guinea pig (*Cavia porcellus*) following ingestion of oxalate containing plants. Can Vet J 2006;47(8):787–9.
[91] Miyamoto Y, Haylor JL, El Nahas AM. Cellular toxicity of catechin analogues containing gallate in opossum kidney proximal tubular (OK) cells. J Toxicol Sci 2004;29(1):47–52.
[92] Degernes LA. Toxicities in waterfowl. Seminars in Avian and Exotic Pet Medicine 1995; 4(1):15–22.
[93] Robens JF, Richard JL. Aflatoxins in animal and human health. Rev Environ Contam Toxicol 1992;127:69–94.
[94] Rauber RH, Dilkin P, Giacomini LZ, et al. Performance of turkey poults fed different doses of aflatoxins in the diet. Poult Sci 2007;86(8):1620–4.
[95] Yegani M, Chowdhury SR, Oinas N, et al. Effects of feeding grains naturally contaminated with *Fusarium* mycotoxins on brain regional neurochemistry of laying hens, turkey poults, and broiler breeder hens. Poult Sci 2006;85(12):2117–23.
[96] Ergün E, Ergün L, Eşsiz D. Light and electron microscopic studies on liver histology in chicks fed aflatoxin. Dtsch Tierarztl Wochenschr 2006;113(10):363–8.
[97] Dvorska JE, Pappas AC, Karadas F, et al. Protective effect of modified glucomannans and organic selenium against antioxidant depletion in the chicken liver due to T-2 toxin-contaminated feed consumption. Comp Biochem Physiol C Toxicol Pharmacol 2007; 145(4):582–7.
[98] Schweitzer SH, Ouist CF, Grimes GL, et al. Aflatoxin levels in corn available as wild turkey feed in Georgia. J Wildl Dis 2001;37(3):657–9.
[99] Young KL, Villar D, Carson TL, et al. Tremorgenic mycotoxin intoxication with penitrem A and roquefortine in two dogs. J Am Vet Med Assoc 2003;222(1):52–3.
[100] Balseiro A, Espí A, Márquez I, et al. Pathological features in marine birds affected by the Prestige's oil spill in the north of Spain. J Wildl Dis 2005;41:371–8.
[101] Oropesa AL, Pérez-López M, Hernández D, et al. Acetylcholinesterase activity in seabirds affected by the Prestige oil spill on the Galician coast (NW Spain). Sci Total Environ 2007; 372(2–3):532–8.
[102] Yamato IG, Maede Y. Hemolytic anemia in wild seaducks caused by marine oil pollution. J Wildl Dis 1996;32:381–4.
[103] Briggs KT, Gershwin ME, Anderson DW. Consequences of petrochemical ingestion and stress on the immune system of seabirds. ICES J Mar Sci 1997;54(4):718–25.

[104] Orbell JD, Ngeh LN, Bigger SW, et al. Whole-bird models for the magnetic cleansing of oiled feathers. Mar Pollut Bull 2004;48(3–4):336–40.

[105] Grossman J. What's hiding under the sink: dangers of household pesticides. Environ Health Perspect 1995;103(6):550–4.

[106] White DH, Seginak JT. Brain cholinesterase inhibition in songbirds from pecan groves sprayed with phosalone and disulfoton. J Wildl Dis 1990;26(1):103–6.

[107] Franson JC, Smith MR. Poisoning of wild birds from exposure to anticholinesterase compounds and lead: diagnostic methods and selected cases. Seminars in Avian and Exotic Pet Medicine 1999;8(1):3–11.

[108] Heatley JJ, Jowett PLH. What is your diagnosis? J Avian Med Surg 2000;14(4):283–4.

[109] Blus LJ, Stroud RK, Sutton GM, et al. Canada goose die-off related to simultaneous application of three anticholinesterase insecticides. Northwest Naturalist 1991;72(1):29–33.

[110] Simsa S, Hasdai A, Dan H, et al. Induction of tibial dyschondroplasia in turkeys by tetramethylthiuram disulfide (thiram). Poult Sci 2007;86(8):1766–71.

[111] Rath NC, Huff WE, Huff GR, et al. Induction of tibial dyschondroplasia by carbamate and thiocarbamate pesticides. Avian Dis 2007;51(2):590–3.

[112] Plumlee KH. Treatment of insecticide poisoning (VET-405). Western Veterinary Conference. Las Vegas, NV; February 8-12, 2004.

[113] Coats JR. Mechanisms of toxic action and structure-activity relationships for organochlorine and synthetic pyrethroid insecticides. Environ Health Perspect 1990;87:255–62.

[114] Garg UK, Pal AK, Jha GJ, et al. Haemato-biochemical and immuno-pathophysiological effects of chronic toxicity with synthetic pyrethroid, organophosphate and chlorinated pesticides in broiler chicks. Int Immunopharmacol 2004;4(13):1709–22.

[115] Lightfoot TL. Organochlorine disaster in Florida—2 years later. J Avian Med Surg 2001; 15(2):138–40.

[116] Eason CT, Murphy EC, Wright GRG, et al. Assessment of risks of brodifacoum to nontarget birds and mammals in New Zealand. Ecotoxicology 2002;11(1):35–48.

[117] Jenkins JR. The anatomy and physiology of avian emergency and critical care. ABVP Annual Conference. Washington, DC; April 29-May 1, 2005.

[118] Thomson AE, Squires EJ, Gentry PA. Assessment of factor V, VII and X activities, the key coagulant proteins of the tissue factor pathway in poultry plasma. Br Poult Sci 2002;43(2): 313–21.

[119] Tarrant KA, Westlake GE. Histological technique for the identification of poisoning in wildlife by the rodenticide calciferol. Bull Environ Contam Toxicol 1984;32(1):175–8.

[120] Johnson GD, Fagerstone KA. Primary and secondary hazards of zinc phosphide to nontarget wildlife: a review of the literature. Bull Environ Contam Toxicol 1994;71:1019–25.

[121] Ozcan K, Ozen H, Karaman M. Nitrosative tissue damage and apoptotic cell death in kidneys and livers of naturally ethylene glycol (antifreeze)-poisoned geese. Avian Pathol 2007;36(4):325–9.

[122] Radi ZA, Miller DL, Thompson LJ. Ethylene glycol toxicosis in chickens. Vet Hum Toxicol 2003;45(1):36–7.

[123] Howard LL, Papendick R, Stalis IH, et al. Fenbendazole and albendazole toxicity in pigeons and doves. J Avian Med Surg 2002;16(3):203–10.

[124] Lightfoot TL. Warning: fenbendazole in cockatiels. Exotic DVM Veterinary Magazine 1999; 1.4:39.

[125] Gartrell BD, Alley MR, Mitchell AH. Fatal levamisole toxicosis of captive kiwi (*Apteryx mantelli*). N Z Vet J 2005;53(1):84–6.

[126] Stahl S, Kronfeld D. Veterinary nutrition of large psittacines. Seminars in Avian and Exotic Pet Medicine 1998;7(3):128–34.

[127] Rajasree S, Umashankar PR, Lal AV, et al. 1,25-dihydroxyvitamin D3 receptor is upregulated in aortic smooth muscle cells during hypervitaminosis D. Life Sci 2002;70(15): 1777–88.

[128] Stanford M. The effect of UV-B lighting supplementation in African grey parrots. Exotic DVM Veterinary Magazine 2004;6(3):29–32.
[129] Preuss SE, Bartels T, Schmidt V, et al. Vitamin A requirements of alipochromatic ('recessive-white') and coloured canaries (*Serinus canaria*) during the breeding season. Vet Rec 2007;160(1):14–9.
[130] Koutsos EA, Tell LA, Woods LW, et al. Adult cockatiels (*Nymphicus hollandicus*) at maintenance are more sensitive to diets containing excess vitamin A than to vitamin A-deficient diets. J Nutr 2003;133(6):1898–902.
[131] Tang KN, Rowland GN, Veltmann JR. Vitamin A toxicity: comparative changes in bone of the broiler and leghorn chicks. Avian Dis 1985;29(2):416–29.
[132] Latshaw JD, Morishita TY, Sarver CF, et al. Selenium toxicity in breeding ring-necked pheasants (*Phasianus colchicus*). Avian Dis 2004;48(4):935–9.
[133] Ji X, Hu W, Cheng J, et al. Oxidative stress on domestic ducks (Shaoxing duck) chronically exposed in a mercury-selenium coexisting mining area in China. Ecotoxicol Environ Saf 2006;64(2):171–7.
[134] Cork SC. Iron storage disease in birds. Avian Pathol 2000;29(1):7–12.
[135] Mete A, van Zeeland YRA, Vaandrager AB, et al. Partial purification and characterization of ferritin from liver and intestinal mucosa of chickens, turtledoves and mynahs. Avian Pathol 2005;34(5):430–4.
[136] Cubas ZS, Godoy SN. Hemochromatosis in toucans. Exotic DVM Veterinary Magazine 2002;4(3):27–8.
[137] Sheppard C, Dierenfeld E. Iron storage disease in birds: speculation on etiology and implications for captive husbandry. J Avian Med Surg 2002;16(3):192–7.
[138] Otten BA, Orosz SE, Auge S, et al. Mineral content of food items commonly ingested by keel-billed toucans (*Ramphastos sulfuratus*). J Avian Med Surg 2001;15(3):194–6.
[139] Mete A, Hendriks HG, Klaren PHM, et al. Iron metabolism in mynah birds (*Gracula religiosa*) resembles human hereditary haemochromatosis. Avian Pathol 2003;32(6): 625–32.
[140] Drews Amber V, Redrobe SP, Patterson-Kane JC. Successful reduction of hepatocellular hemosiderin content by dietary modification in toco toucans (*Ramphastos toco*) with iron-storage disease. J Avian Med Surg 2004;18(2):101–5.
[141] Mandel S, Amit T, Reznichenko L, et al. Green tea catechins as brain-permeable, natural iron chelators-antioxidants for the treatment of neurodegenerative disorders. Mol Nutr Food Res 2006;50(2):229–34.
[142] West GD, Garner MM, Talcott PA. Hemochromatosis in several species of lories with high dietary iron. J Avian Med Surg 2000;15(4):297–301.
[143] McDonald D. Feeding ecology and nutrition of Australian lorikeets. Seminars in Avian and Exotic Pet Medicine 2003;12(4):195–204.

ELSEVIER
SAUNDERS

Vet Clin Exot Anim 11 (2008) 261–282

VETERINARY
CLINICS
Exotic Animal Practice

Raptor Toxicology

Patrick T. Redig, DVM, PhD*,
Lori R. Arent, BS, MS

*The Raptor Center, College of Veterinary Medicine, University of Minnesota,
1920 Fitch Avenue, St. Paul, MN 55108, USA*

Birds of prey (raptors) are high profile predatory birds positioned on the top of the food chain. They consume both vertebrate and invertebrate prey species and occupy both aquatic and terrestrial environments. Due to these factors, along with their wide range of distribution, raptors are receiving increased recognition for their role as biomonitors or sentinels of ecosystem health. They have proven to be exceptional indicators of risk in the area of toxicology.

Birds of prey have demonstrated the negative impact that toxic agents can produce on animal populations and ecosystem dynamics. Due to their feeding habits, raptors are very susceptible to secondary poisoning and bioaccumulation of toxic substances. This is best illustrated by the severe effect of the organochlorine pesticide DDT (1,1,1-trichloro-2,2-bis(p-chlorophenyl)ethane and its metabolite DDE (1,1-dichloro-2,2-bis(p-chlorophenyl)-ethylene had on the populations of American bald eagles (*Haliaeetus leucocephalus*) and peregrine falcons (*Falco peregrinus*). Both species were nearly brought to extinction due to reproductive failure caused by bioaccumulation of this pesticide in their body tissues.

The nationwide ban on DDT and intense recovery efforts aided these species in rebounding from this toxic event. However birds of prey, both wild and captive, continue to be exposed to toxic agents introduced into their environment. Lead; cholinesterase inhibitors, such as organophosphates and carbamates; and anti-coagulant rodenticides, such as brodifacoum, are the most common toxic agents that currently affect the health of wild birds of prey in the United States. For raptors held in captivity, the list of toxic agents extends to include toxic inhalants such as carbon monoxide and polytetrafluoraethylene (Teflon).

* Corresponding author.
E-mail address: redig001@umn.edu (P.T. Redig).

1094-9194/08/$ - see front matter © 2008 Elsevier Inc. All rights reserved.
doi:10.1016/j.cvex.2007.12.004   *vetexotic.theclinics.com*

Lead poisoning

Background

Poisoning by lead ingestion is the most commonmode of intoxication occurring in raptors. Bald eagles (*Haliaeetus leucocephalus*), golden eagles (*Aquila chrysaetos*), and California condors (*Gymnogyps californianus*) are three species in which it is most prevalent, but poisoning can occur in any raptor that is fed or scavenges upon food or prey animals that contain lead residues [1–3]. From studies conducted in children, it is known that lead impairs cognitive and metabolic functions if it is in the body in any amount—that is, there is no threshold effect. Although intoxicated patients may recover to a point where there are no apparent clinical signs, residual subclinical effects consisting of impaired cognition and other neural functions may be irreversible [4].

Sources of lead

For raptors, the sole source of lead exposure derives from lead residues in the tissues of food items that are scavenged or are inadvertently fed to them. Lead may be in one of three forms: 1) biologically incorporated lead in the tissues originating from consumption of lead by the prey, 2) shotgun pellets embedded in tissue from food items dispatched by shotgun or present in the stomach of dabbling ducks or geese that have scavenged spent ammunition from wetland sediments, or 3) lead fragments embedded in tissue and offal of big game animals that have been killed with a lead bullet. A fourth potential source is lead leached from bullet fragments or shotgun pellets that have been embedded in the tissue of a raptor that has been shot.

Experimental evidence has demonstrated that biologically incorporated lead does not constitute a clinically significant source of lead. Custer and colleagues [5] fed kestrels either mice or cockerels that had been fed lead and found no metal accumulation in the kestrels. These data support the hypothesis that the rate of intake did not exceed the ability of the kestrels to either eliminate the lead or sequester it in bone. However, long-term, repeated exposure to biologically incorporated lead in tissues may contribute to the total body lead burden of a raptor and perhaps lower the dose needed to produce toxic signs in an acute exposure.

Lead from projectiles that is embedded in tissues of raptors also does not appear to contribute to the total body burden. Studies conducted on waterfowl in which lead, iron, and bismuth pellets were implanted into breast muscles of game farm mallards showed no erosion or loss of weight over twelve months of implantation [6] Clinical experience at The Raptor Center with projectile-injured birds further supports this lack of effect (P.T. Redig, unpublished data, 2007).

The principal source of lead in raptors is spent ammunition in food items [1–3,7]. Lead ammunition has been banned for waterfowl hunting on all federal refuges and most state owned lands throughout the U.S. since 1991 and in Canada since 1999. However, it may be used still for waterfowl hunting on private lands and it is used also for upland game hunting and rodent shooting (prairie dogs, gophers, ground squirrels, woodchucks) in the U.S. In the case of the latter, carcasses are typically left in the field, which are often scavenged by raptors. Lead ammunition is used also for big game hunting and, in the case of condors and eagles, there is correlation between the incidence of an annual increase in prevalence of lead poisoning and the deer hunting season [1].

There are substantial interspecific and intraspecific variations in susceptibility to lead intoxication [8,9]. Turkey vultures (*Cathartes aura*) are able to survive higher doses of lead than other birds, and red-tailed hawks (*Buteo jamaicensis*) have been observed experimentally to tolerate higher blood lead levels than commonly encountered in eagles; the reasons for this apparent resistance are not known [10,11].

Birds in general, appear to be more resistant to lead poisoning than mammals [12]. Nevertheless, lead is extremely toxic to raptors. Experimental studies of orally-dosed bald eagles showed that intragastric erosion and uptake of between 19–40 mg of lead was lethal to a bald eagle (4–5 kg) in 10–12 days [13]. One number six shot (about the diameter of a #2 pencil lead) contains approximately 150 mg of lead—an amount sufficient to kill 3–5 eagles if ingested [14].

Kinetics of absorption, tissue distribution and toxicity

Once ingested, lead from ammunication is solubilized in the acidic environment of the stomach and absorbed in the small intestine [15]. Absorption of lead in sufficient amounts to cause acute toxicity is favored in diurnal raptors owing to a lower pH in their stomach—approaching 1, compared with psittacines and granivorous birds and even owls whose stomach pH is around 2–4 [16]. Once absorbed, lead binds to red blood cells, and is then distributed to other body compartments. One is a rapid exchange compartment comprised largely of blood and parenchyma of highly perfused organs that comprise about 4% of the total body burden; another compartment is soft tissue, including the nervous system, which has an intermediate rate of exchange and holds about 2% of the body burden; and the last is bone, a compartment with a slow rate of exchange that may hold 94% of the body burden [17]. Hydroxyapatite crystals in bone have a high affinity for lead and much of the body burden of lead is ultimately stored there. Lead levels in the liver and kidney are used to make a diagnosis of lead poisoning on a post mortem basis, while circulating levels of lead are measured in live birds. It is important to note that in sampling blood for lead residues, only a very small amount of the total body burden is being assessed, and this is from a compartment with dynamic exchange kinetics.

The casting mechanism present in raptors may provide a means of shortening exposure as well as affording a means of eliminating lead fragments from the stomach as a mode of treatment. It also confounds detection and diagnosis of lead as the majority of birds presenting with clinical signs of illness do not have lead in the stomach that can be detected radiographically. In one report [18], only 34% of 96 falcons admitted and treated for lead poisoning had radiographically detectable metal fragments or pellets in the stomachs. Hence, preliminary diagnosis is based frequently on history, signalment, and clinical signs.

Most of the cases of clinical lead poisoning appear to be the result of a single acute exposure, although it is not clear whether the bird needs to retain a piece of lead simply overnight or if it must be retained for several days before being cast or passed through the pylorus in order for poisoning to occur. It may also be that ingestion of multiple meals containing small amounts of lead over a period of several days may result in acute intoxication, such as an eagle returning to a lead-contaminated deer carcass over several days such that the rate of ingestion exceeds the rate of clearance from the blood stream by deposition in bone. Many birds have so-called sub-clinical levels of lead that are probably the result of repeated exposures over long periods of time, as no single exposure was sufficient to produce signs of overt toxicity. A single and massive acute exposure may be associated with a rapid and alarmingly high level of lead to be in the blood, but if the lead is cast from the stomach, the blood level can drop precipitously with the bird exhibiting no clinical signs (TRC—clinical observations).

Mechanism(s) of toxicity with lead

Lead binds to sulfhydryl groups in proteins and breaks disulfide bonds that are critical for maintaining proper conformation for biological activity [11,17]. Organ systems that appear to be most affected by lead in birds are: 1) the erythropoietic system, by virtue of denaturing enzymes in the hemoglobin synthetic pathway, notably porphobilinogen synthase (also known as delta amino levulinic acid dehydratase—ALAD) and ferrochelatase—such inhibition causes anemia and accumulation of hemoglobin precursors (delta amino levulinic acid, protoporphyrins—free and zinc bound) [12,19]; 2) the gastrointestinal tract, due to impairment of gastroenteric motility. (In pigeons, lead causes a cyclic AMP-induced relaxation of smooth muscle in the crop [20,21]); and 3) the nervous system inducing principally signs of muscle weakness, seizures, and blindness [12]. In children, lead is known at low levels to interfere with neural pathways involved with cognitive processes—in higher levels lead causes seizures, blindness, and musculoskeletal weakness [4]. Lead also directly causes an increase in red blood cell fragility leading to hemolysis and biliverdinuria and fibrinoid vascular necrosis in various organs that manifests as perivascular hemorrhage [22]. It may also interfere with cardiac conduction—lead poisoned birds have not well described cardiac dysfunction and on post mortem there is in some cases evidence of myocardial necrosis. Also, some recovered birds have poor stamina thought to be associated with cardiac dysfunction (P.T. Redig, unpublished data, 1999). Other nervous system-related effects include progressive demyelination of peripheral nerves [23–25]. Unlike mammals, renal effects are not observed in raptors (P.T. Redig, unpublished data, 2007).

Syndromes and clinical signs

Lead poisoning can be acute, chronic or sub-clinical as follows:

Cases of acute lead poisoning, as typified by the lead-poisoned bald eagles admitted to The Raptor Center annually, present generally in good flesh with one or more of the following signs: weakness in the legs, dull mentally, visual impairment abundant green urine, and biliverdinuria. They are mildly anemic and hypoproteinemic. Patients will often be in extreme respiratory distress. Blood lead levels will range between 1.0 ppm (100 ug/dL) and 4.0 ppm. The typically affected bird will be hock-sitting, staring upward, passing green urates, and breathing very slowly with prolonged, deep inspirations followed by equally long expirations often accompanied by a sibilant, high-pitched sigh. Treatment of these birds with Ca-EDTA and supportive care is usually unsuccessful; those that do survive have poor stamina, possibly related to cardiac muscle damage (P.T. Redig, unpublished data, 1999).

Cases of chronic toxicity, again in bald eagles, are thin to emaciated, weak, have low hematocrits, low total proteins and exhibit crop stasis. They are depressed and biliverdinuric, but do not typically exhibit neurologic signs other than depression. Their blood lead level is in the 0.6 ppm to 1.0 ppm range. These birds have probably been accumulating lead from serial small repeated exposures, finally reaching a state of impairment that renders them unable to forage effectively, hence leading to their state of inanition. With chelation and supportive care, these eagles usually recover.

Cases of subclinical (apparent) toxicity present in various states of body condition and are typically admitted for some other reason—ie, vehicle collision or other trauma. Their lead levels range between 0.4 ppm and 0.6 ppm, and they exhibit few if any signs associated with lead intoxication. On the premise that any amount of lead in the system is harmful, these birds will receive at least one round of chelation therapy to reduce blood levels below 0.2 ppm (20 ug/dL). Current CDC guidelines for lead in children sets the lowest allowable limit at 0.1 ppm.

Diagnosis

A presumptive diagnosis may be made on the basis of history, signalment, and clinical signs and many clinicians will institute chelation therapy based on these indices [17]. The definitive diagnosis of lead poisoning is based on determining the level of lead in a whole blood sample. The most sensitive method for assessment of lead for clinical purposes is atomic absorption spectrophotometry. As this analysis requires sending a sample to a laboratory, a delay of 1–3 days may ensue before results are known. A useful in-house means of blood lead determination is the Lead Care Analyzer (LeadCare

Blood Lead Testing System, ESA Inc., Chelmsford, MA, USA) [18]. This device uses an electrochemical sensor to measure blood in a small quantity of blood. Designed for use in detecting lead in children, it has an upper level of detection of 0.65 ppm (65 ug/dL). In this respect, it doesn't allow measurement of lead in blood of many of the birds with acute toxicities, nonetheless, its upper limit is well into the range of clinical toxicity for raptors.

Because of the frequency with which lead residues are encountered in eagles [1] every eagle admitted to rehabilitation should evaluated for blood lead level at admission. The decision to treat by chelation is triggered at a blood lead level of 0.2 ppm (20 ug/dL) (based on the results from the LeadCare Analyzer) [18] even though clinical signs of lead poisoning may not be apparent at that level. Between 0.2 and 0.6 ppm, treatment is undertaken to reduce total body burden even though specific clinical signs are not apparent—one to two rounds of chelation generally being sufficient to reduce blood levels below 0.2 ppm. Above 0.6 ppm, therapy is aimed at eliminating clinical signs and may require extensive chelation. Blood samples reading above 0.65 ppm (the analyzer simply reads "High") are sent to a laboratory for full analysis. In our experience, the upper limit of blood lead in bald eagles that results in successful treatment is 1.2 ppm using Ca-EDTA therapy (P.T. Redig, unpublished data, 1996). California condors with blood lead levels as high as 6 ppm have been successfully treated (C. Stringfield, LA ZOO, personal communication, 2007); however, in both situations, birds with levels considerably lower have died.

Goals of treatment

The goals of treatment involve the near simultaneous removal of any remaining lead from the stomach by gavage, endoscopic retrieval or gastrotomy [18,26], and the removal of lead from the tissues by chelation as expeditiously as possible. In addition the provision of supportive care for damaged organ systems is important and may include:

- Hematopoietic: blood transfusions, iron dextran
- Gastrointestinal tract: if radio-dense objects are observed, mechanically remove contents that are accessible (crop, stomach) [17,26]; stimulate crop motility with prokinetics (metaclopramide, propulsid)
- Nervous system: if seizuring is present, control with a benzodiazepine tranquilizer, such as diazepam
- Cardiovascular/renal: support adequate perfusion with fluid therapy.
- All systems: reduce lead content by chelation

Chelators

Since the 1950's, the calcium disodium salt of ethylene diaminetetraacetic acid, $CaNa_2EDTA$ (Ca-EDTA), has been the principle mode of treatment of lead poisoning in birds, domestic animals and humans. Forming stable complexes with divalent metal ions, including lead, iron and copper, it quickly increases the urinary excretion of lead. Ca-EDTA appears to be effective only in releasing and binding to lead stored in bone with minimal effect in removing lead from soft tissues [27]. While there are caveats about incidental chelation of zinc, nephrosis, and CNS toxicity arising from transitory increases in blood lead levels following administration of Ca-EDTA [16], none of these are seen to occur in birds even with high levels of Ca-EDTA and prolonged courses of therapy [18]. Ca-EDTA must be administered parentally as absorption from the gastrointestinal tract is poor. Concentrated solutions of Ca-EDTA (eg, 6.6% solution) administered at 35–50 mg/kg yield small volumes that may be administered intramuscularly, although such injections may be painful [17]. Alternatively, it may be diluted in saline and administered subcutaneously (TRC standard operating procedures), especially for prolonged or repeated therapy. Samour and Naldo [18] reported excellent results in treating falcons with lead poisoning with Ca-EDTA (50 mg/kg) in courses of therapy extending out to 23 days. No deleterious effects were noted and blood lead concentrations were reduced by an average of 84% after five days of treatment. Where post-treatment blood levels remained above 20 ug/dL (0.2 ppm), therapy was extended for another five days, again without negative effect.

Other chelators include British Anti-Lewisite (BAL), d-penicillamine (DPA), and meso-2,3-dimercaptosuccinic acid (DMSA). BAL was originally introduced as an antidote to arsenic-based weaponized gas (Lewisite) and later used to treat intoxications associated with organic arsenical drugs used in the treatment of syphilis [28,29]. Subsequently, it was found to be effective in chelating lead. An advantage of BAL compared with Ca-EDTA is its ability to cross the blood brain barrier. However, BAL is unstable, toxic in all but the briefest of treatment durations, and has been shown in laboratory studies to increase the toxicity of lead [28]. It has been phased out in human medicine in favor of DMSA (see below). D-penicillamine, both an oral and parenterally administered chelator, it has significant side effects in human applications and reports of its use in avian species are few [17].

Meso 2,3-dimercaptosuccinic acid (DMSA), a water-soluble derivative of BAL, has proven utility in treating lead poisoning. It is capable of chelating lead from the brain and other soft tissues, does not have the chemical instability and toxic side effects of BAL, and can be administered orally [25,28]. It does not, however, chelate lead from bone. In a study comparing DMSA against Ca-EDTA in lead poisoned cockatiels (*Nymphicus hollandicus*), DMSA produced a more rapid rate of reduction of blood lead levels compared with Ca-EDTA [30]. However, it had a narrow therapeutic index (less than 2-fold) and there were significant problems with regurgitation among treated birds. Survival rates among lead poisoned cockatiels were not different between DMSA and Ca-EDTA treated birds.

In a retrospective analysis among a collection of zoo birds affected by lead poisoning, DMSA was found to be an effective chelator for birds manifesting low to mid-level toxicity [31]. The advantage of oral administration was borne out in this setting as the chelator was simply sprinkled onto food the birds were receiving in their enclosure for a period of 7–10 days. In this study, birds exhibiting neurologic signs were given an initial intramuscular injection of Ca-EDTA in the interest of more rapidly reducing total body lead burden, followed by the course of DMSA at approximately 30 mg/kg b.i.d.

Elsewhere, combination therapy of lead poisoning with Ca-EDTA and DMSA has yielded favorable results that possibly exceed those obtained with either chelator used alone. Degernes and colleagues [26] describe use of Ca-EDTA alone or in combination with DMSA in lead poisoned Trumpeter Swans (*Cygnus buccinator*). Survival rate was 35% with EDTA alone and 50% with combination therapy.

Laboratory studies in rats comparing Ca-EDTA and DMSA indicate an interesting difference in effects. Ca-EDTA was found to chelate lead from all tissues, producing notable reductions in the liver, kidney, and bone, exhibiting a particularly powerful effect on the latter [27]. So much so, that lead liberated from bone during chelation produced a rise in blood lead levels following a single injection of Ca-EDTA with redistribution to the liver and brain [32]. DMSA on the other hand, rapidly reduced lead in liver, kidney, and brain, but not bone. DMSA was capable of rapidly reducing lead in soft tissues and protecting the nervous system from further insult. However, if used alone, it did not remove lead from bone, thereby leaving a depot that could be a source of long-term lead retention and leaching [33]. From a chemical/kinetics point of view, and absence of negative effects from dual treatment, these studies further support the utility of combination therapy with both of these drugs as an improved therapeutic regimen [28].

In summary, both DMSA and Ca-EDTA are suitable chelators for lead poisoned raptors. Ca-EDTA must be administered parenterally, either by intramuscular, intravenous, or subcutaneous routes. It is the most effective agent for chelating lead stored in bone, however, it may cause redistribution of lead to the liver and brain. Notwithstanding this, it has been used effectively by many clinicians for treating avian lead poisoning. DMSA is more effective than Ca-EDTA in removing lead from soft tissues including the brain, and can be administered orally. However it does not remove lead from bone. Cases of low-level lead intoxications (<0.2 ppm) will respond well to orally administered DMSA. Mid-range intoxications without neurologic signs (0.2–0.65 ppm) will respond well to Ca-EDTA. Combination therapy with Ca-EDTA and DMSA would be indicated at higher blood lead levels and has been reported effective in severely intoxicated swans [26].

Dosing and treatment schedule

The established dose for Ca-EDTA is 35–50 mg/kg given b.i.d. or t.i.d. by intramuscular or subcutaneous routes [20,26]. However, higher doses, up to

100 mg/kg, have been used in birds and experimentally in rats without observed ill effect [18,32].

Accurate dosing of DMSA is critical owing to its narrow therapeutic index; 30 mg/kg/day was recommended by various authors [31,33]. Denver and colleagues [30] concluded from their experimental work in cockatiels that DMSA could be safely administered at 40 mg/kg twice daily for at least 21 days, however doses as low as 15 mg/kg have been reported effective [30].

Interrupted treatment schedules for chelation have typically been the standard approach, based on early studies conducted in children. Classical treatment schedule was 3 days on, 2 days off to allow for replenishment of other divalent cations that were chelated by the Ca-EDTA [28] and allow any developing nephrosis to subside. In birds including raptors, clinicians have deviated considerably from this regimen without ill effect. At TRC we typically chelate for five days, followed by a rest period of 2-3 days during which blood lead level is determined as a guide to the need for further treatment. Denver and colleagues [30] recommended chelating for 21 consecutive days with Ca-EDTA alone or in combination with DMSA. Samour [18] presented a graduated treatment schedule in falcons using Ca-EDTA at 100 mg/kg wherein birds at < 0.3 ppm blood lead received Ca-EDTA for 2 days, while those with 0.3–0.4 ppm blood lead received treatment for four days, and birds between 0.4 and 0.65 ppm blood lead received five days of treatment. Above that level, five days of consecutive treatment followed by one or more repeated schedules was used until the blood lead concentration was reduced below 0.2 ppm. Other authors have confirmed our experience in not encountering problems with prolonged administration of Ca-EDTA (out to 23 days) and at doses up to 100 mg/kg bid [18,30].

Adjuncts to chelation therapy

In addition to fluid therapy, nutritional and supportive care, there may be clinical advantage to anti-oxidative therapy with vitamin C and zinc, as there is evidence that lead is an inducer of free-radicals [29]. Administration of B-vitamin complex may aid the recovery of injury to the nervous system.

Prognosis

Most information about treating lead poisoning in raptors comes from clinical experiences with eagles and condors. These two differ considerably in their tolerance of lead. The upper limit of "treatable" lead poisoning in bald eagles is a blood level of 1.2 ppm, while condors have been treated successfully up to 6 ppm (Stringfield, personal communication). It is likely that other species have their own upper limits, but little data exist from clinical cases to establish these values.

Above the upper threshold limit, death or severe, permanent impairment is the likely outcome, hence euthanasia is most often chosen. Since the kinetics of lead are dynamic there are those few cases that present with levels well above the upper limit that appear to be only mildly affected. They may be a consideration for treatment if in the judgment of the clinician the exposure is thought to be peracute with the expectation that the blood levels will recede rapidly.

Post treatment aspects

Among birds that have survived severe lead toxicity and treatment, there is an unquantifiable chance that some will have permanent damage. The overt expressions of these may include visual impairment and lack of stamina. There is accumulating long-term data among condors that have been treated for lead poisoning that they may successfully repatriate when released, but long-term survivability and productivity has not yet been established. Similarly, such information is also lacking for bald eagles despite many years of treatment and release of recovered birds.

Cholinesterase inhibitors

The two most common groups of cholinesterase (ChE)-inhibiting substances affecting raptors are organophosphates and carbamates. Throughout the world, these toxic agents are used to control pests in the agricultural industry, on golf courses, in domestic applications such as home gardening and landscape maintenance, and in veterinary medicine for parasite control on livestock [34,35]. Their application is often relatively localized and they are short lived in the environment; thus they have a low potential for bioaccumulation, but a high potential for acute toxicity. Based on LD_{50} values for these chemicals, birds are 10%–20% more susceptible to the toxic effects of ChE-inhibiting compounds than mammals [36].

Mechanism of toxicity

Organophosphate and carbamate compounds bind to acetylcholinesterase (AChE), one of several cholinesterases (B-esterase enzymes) in the peripheral and central nervous system. AChE rapidly degrades the neurotransmitter acetylcholine (ACh) and when its catalytic activity is inhibited, ACh accumulates in cholinergic synapses causing cholinergic hyperstimulation of end organs that express muscarinic cholinergic receptors (eg, heart, airways) and initial contraction, followed by paralysis of skeletal muscles, which possess nicotinic cholinergic receptors [37]. The major toxic effect of these chemicals is compromised cardiopulmonary function (ie, reduced ventilation due to excessive secretions and bronchoconstriction, bradycardia progressing to asystole, and paralysis of voluntary muscles of respiration) One major difference between the two groups of inhibitors is that organophosphate compounds bind irreversibly to AChE, while carbamates may separate from

AChE via hydrolytic removal, allowing for reactivation of the enzyme. In addition to neural acetylcholinesterase, ChE inhibitors can inhibit the activity of butyrylcholinesterase ("non-specific" cholinesterase) in blood serum.

Based on literature review, diazinon (0,0-diethyl-0-(2-isopropyl-6-methyl-pyrimidine-4-yl), fenthion (0,0-dimethyl 0-[3-methyl-4-(methylthio)phenyl] phosphorothioate); monocrotophos (Dimethyl (E)-1-methyl-2 (methyl carbamoyl) vinyl phosphate); and famphur (4-dimethozyphosphinothioyloxy-N,N-dimtthylbenzenefonamide) are the most common organophosphate compounds reported in raptor species in the United States. The main carbamate reported is carbofuran (2,3 dihydro-2,2-dimethyl-7-benzofuranyl methylcarbamate).

Exposure

Birds of prey are poisoned by ChE inhibitors in two major ways. They can either ingest the poison directly by scavenging on carcasses treated with these products or succumb to secondary poisoning from ingesting intoxicated prey [34,38,39]. One particularly interesting case involved tertiary poisoning of a great horned owl (*Bubo virginianus*). This owl fed on a red-tailed hawk (*Buteo jamaicencis*) that died following ingestion of a black-billed magpie (*Pica pica*) that obtained famphur from the hair of dusted cattle [34].

Mass die-offs of raptors due to exposure to ChE-inhibiting toxic agents have been reported [38,40,41]. Species which roost communally during the non-breeding season or migrate to more favorable climates and congregate in suitable wintering areas are more vulnerable to the effects of toxic agents. In 1995, this was demonstrated in Argentina, where a large population of Swainson's hawks (*Buteo swainsoni*) winters in the pampas and feeds on insects in agricultural areas. Sunflower crops were sprayed with monocrotophos for pest control and the birds fed on poisoned insects, resulting in a die off of over 20,000 hawks (estimated 5% of the world's Swainson's hawk population) during one wintering season [40].

Diagnosis

Due to the acute toxicity of ChE inhibitors, diagnosis of organophosphate or carbamate poisoning is often made post-mortem. However, because these compounds produce biochemical changes but no gross or macroscopic lesions, and they break down quickly in dead animals, diagnosis can be challenging. Stomach contents are analyzed for the presence of the toxic compounds, and levels of insecticide residues in liver, kidney, fat, and brain tissues are measured using gas chromatography [39]. Definitive diagnosis, however, is often made by measuring ChE activity in the brain; however, this does not identify the specific type of toxin involved. Cholinesterase activity is commonly measured using either the electrometric method [42], that measures change in assay pH as a function of ChE activity, or a modified version of Ellman's calorimetric method [43,44], measuring light absorbance. A 20% decrease in plasma activity is indicative of exposure; a 50% or greater decrease is considered diagnostic for cholinesterase inhibitor exposure [44].

For those individuals recovered alive following ingestion of the poison, diagnosis can be made by assessing clinical symptoms and analyzing the plasma for activity of cholinesterases. This activity is most often measured as a composite of cholinesterases including AChE, butyrylcholinesterase (BChE) and carboxylesterase (CbE), not solely AChE. In birds of prey, clinical symptoms often include central nervous system effects such as ataxia, convulsions, lethargy, protrusion of the nictitans, a non-responsive attitude, and respiratory distress; peripheral nicotinic effects such as clenched feet and paralysis; and peripheral muscarinic effects such as increased salivary secretions, crop/GI stasis and regurgitation, and bradycardia [45]. In bald eagles (*Haliaeetus leucocephalus*), the heart rate can drop from a normal resting rate of 180-200 beats per minute to as low as 60-80 beats per minute (The Raptor Center, unpublished data, 1992). Levels of plasma ChE activity are measured using the same assays as for brain ChE activity; however, one complication is that relatively few normal plasma values have been identified for different species of raptors (Table 1). Thus, testing may also involve submitting a normal sample from a conspecific bird for comparison. When death occurs, it is usually from respiratory failure [50].

Treatment

In raptors, treatment is initiated based on clinical signs and suspicion of AChE inhibition, as lab results may take 1-5 days to confirm the diagnosis. Unfortunately, in most cases, the exact causative agent is unknown so a general treatment plan is initiated. First, to decrease absorption of remaining toxic agents in the gastrointestinal tract, any crop contents present (hawks, falcons, eagles, vultures, osprey) must be manually removed, and activated charcoal (2-8 mg/kg; 1g diluted in 5cc water) administered orally BID until the GI tract has cleared.

In addition, treatment includes administering atropine sulfate, 0.5 mg/kg. This can be repeated TID-QID if severe bradycardia persists; one fourth of the dose can be given intravenously (IV) for rapid uptake and delivery, and the rest intramuscularly (IM). Atropine, a parasympatholytic drug, is a competitive muscarinic receptor antagonist and will interrupt the actions of acetylcholine on the heart, airways, gut and other end organs. In the heart for example, it will elevate sinus rate and improve atrioventricular conduction. It will also generally decrease secretions (mouth, digestive system, respiratory system) and decreasing the motility of the GI tract, often causing stasis in birds. Atropine is not effective at nicotinic cholinergic receptor sites and thus will not mitigate skeletal muscle paralysis induced by toxic ChE inhibitors.

Pralidoxime iodide (2-PAM) is an antidote for organophosphate poisoning in mammals, but has shown mixed results in raptors. One study reported that

Table 1
Normal brain and plasma ChE levels recorded in raptor species

Species	Brain ChE[a] micromoles acetylthiocholine hydrolyzed/min/gm wet weight brain tissue	Plasma ChE Micromoles/min/ml unless otherwise indicated
Bald eagle (*Haliaeetus leucocephalus*)	16.0 [44,46]	0.17 ΔpH/hr (n = 6; range 0.16–0.19) [47]
Golden eagle (*Aquila chrysaetos*)	16.0 [44] 14 [46]	–
Peregrine falcon (*Falco peregrinus*)	18.6 [44]	0.13 ΔpH/hr (n = 3; range 0.12–0.14) [47]
Red-tailed hawk (*Buteo jamaicensis*)	17.5 [44], 19 [46]	0.566–1.009 [48] 0.22 ΔpH/hr (n = 6; range 0.17–0.28) [47]
Sharp-shinned hawk (*Accipiter striatus*)	21.5 [44], 21 [46]	–
Great horned owl (*Bubo virginianus*)	15.5 [44], 16 [46]	0.406–0.459 [49]
Eastern screech owl (*Megascops asio*)	18.7 [44], 19 [46]	–
Spotted owl (*Strix occidentalis*)	14.6 [44]	–
Cooper's hawk (*Accipiter cooperii*)	24 [46]	–
American kestrel (*Falco sparverius*)	27 [46]	–
Common barn owl (*Tyto alba*)	20 [46]	0.623 [37]
Northern goshawk (*Accipiter gentilis*)	–	0.231 [37]
European kestrel (*Falco tinnunculus*)	–	0.831 [37]
Tawny owl (*Strix aluco*)	–	0.205 [37]
European sparrowhawk (*Accipiter nisus*)	–	0.555 [37]
Marsh harrier (*Circus aeruginosus*)	–	0.222 [37]

Abbreviation: ChE, cholinesterase.
[a] Brain levels are a composite measure of both ChE and butyrylcholinesterase.

a dose of 100 mg/kg given IM within 24 hours of exposure to monocrotophos was effective in recovering individuals from several different species in Israel [51]. Other sources indicated that 20 mg/kg 2-PAM was sufficient to break the organophosphate/AChE bond but that higher doses may actually reduce AChE activity. In addition, 2-PAM has been shown to be contraindicated in the treatment of some carbamate ChE inhibitors, such as carbaryl, as it further inhibits AChE activity [52]. Thus, unless the toxic agent is positively identified as an organophosphate and the patient recovered quickly after exposure, 2-PAM should not be included in a general treatment protocol.

In addition to treatments which target the direct effects of the toxic agent, supportive therapy should be initiated to maintain the nutritional and hydration needs of the patient (Table 2).

Data from the raptor center

Over the past 10 years (1998–2007), The Raptor Center has measured plasma ChE levels in 59 raptors. This included 49 bald eagles, 3 peregrine falcons, and 7 red-tailed hawks. Samples were analyzed by the Veterinary Diagnostic Lab, College of Veterinary Medicine, University of Minnesota, using the electrometric assay that reports ChE activity as a change (delta) in pH units per hour [42].

Of 49 samples from bald eagles, six were taken from clinically normal birds and the average ChE level was delta 0.17 pH units per hour. In the 43 remaining samples, 22 showed a 20% reduction in activity (0.10–0.14), and 21 showed a 50% or greater reduction (0.03-0.09). Twelve of the birds showing a 20% reduction in enzyme activity were admitted due to traumatic injuries; routine testing discovered the suppression in enzymatic activity. Six of the birds with a 50% reduction in enzyme activity also had traumatic injuries; the remaining 15 were admitted only with symptoms of toxicity. Clinical presentation varied in these cases, and there did not appear to be a correlation between the symptoms exhibited, including bradycardia, and the degree to which ChE activity was inhibited.

In summary, the morbidity and mortality produced by ChE-inhibiting compounds in wild raptors is unknown. Limited recovery of intoxicated birds, the lack of reference values for "normal" brain and plasma cholinesterase activities in different raptor species, and limited testing on individuals

Table 2
Supportive therapy for daily maintenance in raptor species

Daily fluid maintenance	50 cc/kg/day lactated Ringers administered IV, SQ, IO, PO; divided into BID treatments
Replenishment of fluid deficit	Administered in addition to maintenance over a 48–72 hour period; for example, the fluid deficit for a 1 kg raptor estimated to be 10% dehydrated = 100cc.
Decrease gastric mucosa damage	Zantac (ranitidine) 0.2–0.5 mg/kg IM BID
Daily caloric requirement—Bird in good to fair body condition with GI motility evident	250 kcal/kg/day in the form of easily digestible meat (no fur, feathers, bones); can be administered SID or divided into BID feedings
Daily caloric requirement—Bird in poor body condition	250 kcal/kg/day in a slurry gavaged directly into the stomach; volume to be divided into BID or TID treatments depending on patient tolerance. Carnivore Care (Oxbow Company) recommended.
External warmth	Incubator set at 80°F (26.7°C)

Abbreviations: BID, twice daily; IO, intraosseous; IM, intramuscular; IV, intravenous; PO, orally; SID, once daily; SQ, subcutaneously; TID, three times daily.

recovered with traumatic injuries have hindered an assessment of the importance of anticholinesterase toxicity in raptors.

Anti-coagulant rodenticides

In the United States, there are nine registered rodenticides currently un-
dergoing a risk assessment for human and ecosystem health (EPA, 2007).
Rodenticides are widely used to control rodent populations both by the
general public for home use, as well as by commercial operations such as
orchards; thus they are used in both urban and rural areas [53,54]. Rodents
considered pests include rats, mice, gophers, moles, chipmunks, ground
squirrels, muskrats, and mongoose, many of which are common prey species
for raptors. Rabbits, opossums, and other mammal species are also tar-
geted. Rodenticides with an anti-coagulant mode of action are especially
toxic to raptors and their lethal affects have been well documented.

Warfarin, the first anti-coagulant rodenticide synthesized, is a coumarin-
based product that has a short biological half life and requires chronic
exposure to elicit fatal effects. Many rodent species developed resistance
to it and in response, compounds with greater physiologic persistence,
such as bromadiolone and brodifacoum, were produced. As rodents cannot
eliminate these products by vomiting, anticoagulants can kill a rodent in
a single feeding. Brodifacoum (3-[3-(4′-bromobiphenly-4-yl)-1,2,3,4-tetrahy-
dro-1-naphthyl]-=4-hydroxycoumarin) is the most frequently used anticoagulant rodenticide on the world market today [55]. In the U.S. its use is
prohibited in open fields but permitted in and around structures [56]. It is
the main toxic agent found in rodent baits with several trade names including D-Con, Talon, and Havoc and will be the main focus of this discussion.

Mechanism of toxic activity

Brodifacoum is a second generation anticoagulant rodenticide (SGAR),
sometimes referred to as a "superwarfarin rodenticide." Most often, it is
absorbed through the GI tract, although it can also be absorbed through the
skin and respiratory system. Its direct toxic effect is to interfere with the vitamin
K epoxide reductase cycle, thus slowly decreasing the amount of active vitamin
K in the blood. Vitamin K is necessary for the synthesis of clotting factors such
as prothrombin [57]. In addition, brodifacoum attacks the blood capillaries, increasing their permeability and causing slow persistent internal hemorrhage that
leads to shock and death. Like other SGARs, brodifacoum is lipolytic in nature
and binds tightly to membranes, resulting in slow urinary elimination [58]. A single dose of brodifacoum will usually result in rodent death in 4 to 5 days.

Exposure

For rodent control, brodifacoum bait is available either as ready-to-use
blue or green cereal-based pellets or an extruded block, both containing

0.02-0.05 mg brodifacoum/g of bait material. Raptors, like many other non-target predators and scavengers, are exposed to brodifacoum via secondary poisoning. As of November 2006, the EPA received SGAR incident reports on 18 species of raptors primarily from New York and California. Seven species of owls (103 individuals) and eleven species of diurnal birds (135 individuals) comprised the list and brodifacoum was the rodenticide detected in 87% of reported exposures [59].

EPA reports of SGAR residue detection in raptors [22]
    Owls
        71 Great horned owls (*Bubo virginianus*)
        18 Eastern screech owls (*Megascops asio*)
        8 Common barn owls (*Tyto alba*)
        2 Northern spotted owls (*Strix occidentalis*)
        2 Long-eared owls (*Asio otus*)
        1 Barred owl (*Strix varia*)
        1 Northern saw-whet owl (*Aegolis acadicus*)
    Diurnal Raptors
        85 Red-tailed hawks (*Buteo jamaicensis*)
        24 Cooper's hawks (*Accipiter cooperii*)
        13 Golden eagles (*Aquila chrysaetos*)
        2 Bald eagles (*Haliaeetus leucocephalus*)
        3 Red-shouldered hawks (*Buteo lineatus*)
        2 Sharp-shinned hawks (*Accipiter striatus*)
        1 Broad-winged hawk (*Buteo platypterus*)
        2 American kestrels (*Falco sparverius*)
        1 Unidentified hawk
        1 Turkey vulture (*Cathartes aura*)
        1 Black vulture (*Coragyps atratus*)

In rodents, several days elapse between initial rodenticide ingestion and the fatal hemorrhage; thus they often return to the bait for multiple "meals," accumulating the level of toxin in their system [56]. Not only does the time delay increase the probability of an intoxicated rodent being preyed upon, it also presents the predator with a higher dose of toxin that approaches or reaches its LD_{50}. In addition, unlike their first generation counterparts (such as warfarin), SGARs are only slowly metabolized by the liver, thus allowing predators to accumulate lethal doses by ingesting multiple intoxicated rodents. The LD_{50} value reported for rats is 0.27-0.3 mg/kg b.w; for mice 0.4 mg/kg b.w. The LD_{50} for bird species ranges from <0.75 mg/kg (Canada goose, *Branta canadensis*) to >20 mg/kg (Paradise shelduck, *Tadorna variegata*) [60].

Animals can carry sublethal levels of brodifacoum. In the case of wild raptors, it is possible that exposure predisposes them to events such as predation, traumatic injuries, and reduced hunting ability. Thus, mortality can occur indirectly from exposure to these toxic agents and therefore the full impact of rodenticide use for raptors is not realized.

Diagnosis

Similar to diagnosing toxicosis due to ChE inhibitors, raptor intoxication due to rodenticides is often discovered post mortem. Diagnosis is made by testing the liver for rodenticide residues using high performance liquid chromatography [61]. In mammals, ante-mortem diagnosis of anticoagulant exposure involves measuring the hematocrit, clotting parameters such as prothrombin time, and rodenticide residues in the blood or liver.

For a free-ranging bird presented with little recovery information, diagnosis is often made based entirely on clinical signs at the time of presentation. Raptors that have ingested brodifacoum often show pallor of mucous membranes and a marked anemia in the absence of any traumatic injury (normal packed cell volume (PCV) for most raptor species falls within the range of 35%–50% [62]). In addition, they are weak, quiet, and frequently have subcutaneous ecchymoses, especially over the abdomen [63]. They bleed profusely from superficial wounds such as abrasions and punctures, eg, venipuncture.

Treatment

To treat a raptor exhibiting symptoms of SGAR toxicity, any toxin remaining in the digestive tract must be cleared. Thus, crop contents must be manually removed and stomach contents neutralized by lavage with activated charcoal (2-8 mg/kg; 1g diluted in 5cc water). Vitamin K_1 (2.2 mg/kg q4-8 hrs) should be administered IM until the bird is stable; then q24 orally for a minimum of 3 weeks until body systems return to normal function [64]. In mammals, prothrombin time is used to monitor clotting activity and follow recovery of a poisoned patient; in birds, little information regarding clotting profiles is available and thus they are not reliable parameters to diagnosis or monitor an intoxicated patient [65].

If the patient presents with a PCV less than 20%, or if during treatment the PCV drops below 20%, the blood loss can be treated with a transfusion from a healthy, conspecific individual. This will help support the patient for a few days until its system is regenerating a sufficient number of red blood cells on its own. A safe volume to remove and administer is 1% of the bird's body weight. Thus, a healthy 1000 g red-tailed hawk can safely donate 10 cc blood and a 1000 g recipient can accept this volume as a bolus injection. To prevent additional blood loss, the intraosseous (ulna or tibiotarsus) mode of administration is recommended.

In addition to replacing blood loss and clotting factors, supportive care should be initiated (Table 1). Whenever a clinician is handling and managing a bird suffering from intoxication with a rodenticide, care must be taken to prevent self-inflicted trauma and subsequent hemorrhage.

Raptor center data

Over the past 10 years, The Raptor Center has admitted 7462 raptors, primarily from Minnesota and surrounding Midwestern states. None of these patients had evidence of SGAR coagulopathy indicative of rodenticide toxicity. However, in post-mortem evaluations of patients dying from other causes, brodifacoum residues were commonly identified in great horned owls and red-tailed hawks (Arno Wunschmann,Veterinary Diagnostic Lab, College of Veterinary Medicine, University of MN, personal communication).

Inhaled toxins

Birds have an efficient respiratory system that is extremely sensitive to airborne particles. Thus, pet birds have to rely on their caretakers to provide adequate ventilation at all times and reduce exposure to potentially fatal gases and fumes. Maintaining a raptor in captivity requires the same vigilance. Most captive raptors are housed in outdoor facilities that meet state and federal guidelines. However, for eyases (unfledged nestlings) raised indoors, training purposes, or travel, raptors can be housed in indoor enclosed environments and are highly susceptible to the effects of airborne toxins. Polytetrafluoroethylene (PTFE) and carbon monoxide are two of the potentially hazardous compounds that should be monitored carefully if raptors are housed indoors.

Polytetrafluoroethylene (PTFE)

Teflon, the brand name of PTFE, is a nonstick coating used on many products including cookware, drip pans, and heat bulbs. When these products are heated above 280°C (536°F), the PTFE coating is unstable and toxic fumes (carbonyl fluoride, perfluoroisobutylene, and hydrogen fluoride) are released by a process called pyrolysis [66]. If normal cooking practices are followed, the temperature of cookware does not reach this temperature limit and it is safe to use. However, if a PTFE-coated pan is allowed to boil dry, an unfilled pan is heated on high, or the PTFE coating has become damaged, toxic particles and fumes can be released. PTFE-coated drip pans are highly hazardous and should not be used at all in a household with birds. The pans, located under burners, will reach over 600°F or higher within minutes during normal use because of their close proximity to the heating element of the burner.

Some brands of heating lamps are also coated with PTFE to protect them and make them easy to clean. As the bulbs warm, toxic fumes can be released and cause mortality in birds. Incidents of raptors killed due to toxicity from Teflon-coated heat bulbs has been reported [67].

The toxic fumes released by overheated teflon cause severe edematous pneumonia. Blood capillaries in the lungs hemorrhage and the lungs fill with fluid and blood leading to acute respiratory distress and most commonly death. If a bird has been affected by PTFE, it is often off its perch, uncoordinated, open mouth breathing with respiratory rails, and will bob its tail with each respiratory effort [63].

Teflon toxicity is usually acute and fatal. However, if a bird suffers from mild exposure and is recovered quickly, treatment includes providing humidified oxygen, diuretics to reduce pulmonary edema, non-steroidal anti-inflammatory drugs, broad-spectrum antibiotics, and supportive care [63] (Table 1).

Carbon monoxide

Another inhalant toxic to birds is carbon monoxide (CO). Like people, birds can be exposed to hazardous levels of CO if housed in an area with a faulty working furnace, or if confined in an operating vehicle with poor ventilation and/or leaks in its exhaust system. CO does not directly harm the lungs or lung capillaries, rather it decreases the oxygen carrying capacity of hemoglobin [62,63]. In pet birds, symptoms include dyspnea, ataxia, depression, and nausea. CO poisoning in raptors is most often fatal, as the exposure is not immediately realized. Harris's hawks (*Buteo unicinctus*) seem to be extremely sensitive to CO and exposure has been implicated in several deaths during travel. The birds that died were housed in travel containers (giant hoods) in the enclosed bed of pick-up trucks.

Miscelleneous inhalants

In addition to concerns surrounding Teflon and carbon monoxide, other household compounds can cause respiratory illness in raptors. Bleach (used for disinfecting travel crates and housing structures), naphthalene (often used to store spare feathers for imping—feather replacement—purposes), tobacco smoke, and some disinfectant sprays can cause varying degrees of respiratory illness, depending on the circumstances of exposure [62]. Good management practices must be employed to house raptors in well ventilated areas and limit exposure to potentially toxic inhalants.

Acknowledgment

The authors express sincere appreciation to Dr. David Brown for his critical review of this manuscript.

References

[1] Kramer JL, Redig PT. Sixteen years of lead poisoning in eagles—1980–1995: an epizootiologic view. J Raptor Res 1997;31:327–32.
[2] Miller MJR, Wayland E, Dzus EH, et al. Availability and ingestion of lead shotshell pellets by migrant bald eagles in Saskatchewan. J Raptor Res 2000;34:167–74.

[3] Pattee OH, Bloom PH, Scott JM, et al. Lead hazards within the range of the California Condor. Condor 1990;92:931–7.

[4] Needleman H. Lead poisoning. Annu Rev Med 2004;55:209–22.

[5] Custer TW, Franson JC, Pattee OH. Tissue lead distribution and hematologic effects in American Kestrels (Falco sparverius L.) fed biologically incorporated lead. J Wildl Dis 1984;20(1):39–43.

[6] Sanderson GC, Anderson WL, Foley GL, et al. Effects of lead, iron, and bismuth alloy shot embedded I the breast muscles of game-farm mallards. J Wildl Dis 1998;34:688–97.

[7] Church ME, Gwiazda R, Risebrough RW, et al. Ammunition is the principal source of lead accumulated by california condors re-introduced to the wild. Environ Sci Technol 2006; 40(19):6143–50, Ammunition is the principal source of lead for condors.

[8] Reiser MH, Temple SA. Effects of chronic lead ingestion on birds of prey. In: Cooper JE, Greenwood AG, editors. Recent advances in the study of raptor diseases. Keighley (England): Chiron Publications Ltd; 1981. p. 21–5.

[9] Beyer WN, Spann JW, Sileo L, et al. Lead poisoning in six captive avian species. Arch Environ Contam Toxicol 1988;17:121–30.

[10] Carpenter JW, Pattee OH, Fritts SH, et al. Experimental lead poisoning in turkey vultures (Cathartes aura). J Wildl Dis 2003;39:95–104.

[11] Redig PT, Lawler EM, Schwartz S, et al. Effects of chronic exposure to sublethal concentrations of lead acetate on heme synthesis and immune function in Red-tailed Hawks. Arch Environ Contam Toxicol 1991;21:72–7.

[12] Lumeij S. Clinicopathologic aspects of lead poisoning in birds: a review. Vet Q 1985;7:133–8.

[13] Pattee O, Wiemeyer SN, Mulhern BM, et al. Experimental leadshot poisoning in bald eagles. J Wildl Manage 1981;45:806–10.

[14] Fry M. Assessment of lead contamination sources exposing California Condors. Species Conservation and Recovery Program Reports, 2003–02. Sacramento: California Department of Fish and Game, Habitat Conservation Planning Branch; 2003.

[15] Fisher IJ, Pain DJ, Thomas VG. A review of lead poisoning from ammunition sources in terrestrial birds. Biol Conserv 2006;131:421–32.

[16] Duke GE. Alimentary canal: secretion and digestion, special digestive functions, and absorption. In: Sturkie PD, editor. Avian physiology. 4th edition. New York: Springer-Verlag; 1986. p. 289–302.

[17] Mautino M. Lead and zinc intoxication in zoological medicine: a review. J Zoo Wildl Med 1997;28:28–35.

[18] Samour JH, Naldo J. Diagnosis and therapeutic management of lead toxicosis in falcons in Saudi Arabia. J Avian Med Surg 2002;16(1):16–20.

[19] Hoffman DJ, Patee OH, Wiemeyer SN, et al. Effects of lead shot ingestion on delta-aminolevulinic acid dehydratase activity, hemoglobin concentration, and serum chemistry in bald eagles. J Wildl Dis 1981;17(3):423–31.

[20] Corey-Slechta DA, Garman RH, Seidman D. Lead induced crop dysfunction in the pigeon. Toxicol Appl Pharmacol 1980;52:426–7.

[21] Boyer IJ, DiStefano V. An investigation of the mechanism of lead-induced relaxation of pigeon crop smooth muscle. J Pharmacol Exp Ther 1985;234:616–23.

[22] Ochiai IK, Jin K, Itakura C, et al. Pathological study of lead poisoning in Whooper Swans (Cygnus cygnus) in Japan. Avian Dis 1992;36:313–23.

[23] Hunter B, Haigh JC. Demyelinating peripheral neuropathy in a guinea hen associated with subacute lead intoxication. Avian Dis 1978;22:344–9.

[24] Hunter B, Wobeser G. Encephalopathy and peripheral neuropathy in lead-poisoned Mallard Ducks. Avian Dis 1980;24:169–78.

[25] Platt SR, Helmick KE, Graham J, et al. Peripheral neuropathy in a turkey vulture with lead toxicosis. J Am Vet Med Assoc 1999;214:1218–20.

[26] Degernes LA, RK Frank, Freeman ML, et al. Lead poisoning in trumpeter swans. Proceedings of the Annual Meeting of the Association of Avian Veterinarians, Seattle, WA; 1989. p. 144–155.

[27] Hammond PB, Aronson AL, Olson WC. The mechanism of mobilization of lead by ethylenediaminetetraacetate. J Pharmacol Exp Ther 1967;157:196–206.

[28] Andersen O. Principles and recent developments in chelation treatment of metal intoxication. Chem Rev 1999;99:2683–710.

[29] Gurer H, Ercal N. Can antioxidants be beneficial in the treatment of lead poisoning? Free Radic Biol Med 2000;29:927–45.

[30] Denver MC, Tell LA, Galey FD, et al. Comparison of two heavy metal chelators for treatment of lead toxicosis in cockatiels. Am J Vet Res 2000;61:935–40.

[31] Hoogesteijn AL, Raphael BL, Calle P, et al. Oral treatment of avian lead intoxication with meso-2,3dimercaptosuccinic acid. J Zoo Wildl Med 2003;34:82–7.

[32] Cory-Slechta DA, Weiss B, Cox C. Mobilization and redistribution of lead over the course of calcium disodium ethylenediamine tetraacetate chelation therapy. J Pharmacol Exp Ther 1987;243:804–13.

[33] Corey-Slechta DA. Mobilization of lead over the course of DMSA chelation therapy and long-term efficacy. J Pharmacol Exp Ther 1988;246:84–91.

[34] Henny CJ, Kolbe EJ, Hill EF, et al. Case history of bald eagles and other raptors killed by organophosphorous insecticides topically applied to livestock. J Wildl Dis 1987;23:292–5.

[35] Kwan Y. Pesticide poisoning events in wild birds in Korea from 1998–2002. J Wildl Dis 2004.

[36] Humphreys DJ. Veterinary toxicology. 3rd edition. London: Baillere Tindall; 1988. p. 179–82.

[37] Roy C. Plasma B-esterase activities in European raptors. J Wildl Dis 2005;41(1):184–208.

[38] Hill EF, Mendenhall WM. Secondary poisoning of Barn owls with Famphur, an organophosphate insecticide. J Wildl Manage 1980;44:676–81.

[39] Reece RL, Handson P. Observations on the accidental poisoning of birds by organophosphate insecticides and other toxic substances. Vet Rec 1982;111:453–5.

[40] Goldstein MI, Lacher TE Jr, woodbridge B, et al. Monocrotophos-induced mass mortality of Swainson's hawks in Argentina, 1995–1996. Ecotoxicology 1999;8:201–14.

[41] Mendenhall VM, Paz U. Mass mortality of birds of prey caused by azodrin, an organophosphate insecticide. Biol Conserv 1977;11:163–70.

[42] Mohammad FK, Al-Baggou BK, Alias AS, et al. Application of an electrometric method for measurement of in vitro inhibition of blood cholinesterases from sheep, goats and cattle by dichlorvos and carbaryl. Vet Med 2006;51(2):45–50.

[43] Ellman GI, Courtney KD, Andres V Jr, et al. A new and rapid colorimetric determination of cholinesterase activity. Biochem Pharmacol 1961;7:88–95.

[44] Hill EF, Flemming WJ. Anticholinesterase poisoning of birds: field monitoring and diagnosis of acute poisoning. Environ Toxicol Chem 1982;1:27–38.

[45] Dumonceaux G, Harrison GJ. Toxins. In: Ritchie BW, Harrison GJ, Harrison LR, editors. Avian medicine principles and applications. Lake Worth (FL): Wingers Publishing; 1994. p. 1049–51.

[46] Hill EF. Brain cholinesterase activity of apparently normal wild birds. J Wildl Dis 1988; 24(1):55–61.

[47] Veterinary Diagnostic Laboratory, University of Minnesota, College of Veterinary Medicine.

[48] Porter S. Pesticide poisoning in birds of prey. In: Redig PT, Cooper JE, Remple JD, et al, editors. Raptor biomedicine. Minneapolis: University of MN Press; 1993. p. 239–45.

[49] Buck JA, Brewer LW, Hooper MJ, et al. Monitoring great horned owls for pesticide exposure in South central IA. J Wildl Manage 1996;60(2):321–31.

[50] Storm JE, Rozman KK, Doull J. Occupational exposure limits for 30 organophosphate pesticides based on inhibition of red blood cell acetylcholinesterase. Toxicology 2000;105: 1–29.

[51] Shlosberg A. Treatment of monocrotophos-poisoned birds of prey with pralidoxamine iodide. J Am Vet Med Assoc 1976;169(9):989–90.

[52] Meerdink GL. Organophosphorous and carbamate insecticide poisoning. In: Kirk RW, editor. Current Veterinary Therapy. vol. 10. Philadelphia: W.B. Saunders; 1989. p. 135–7.

[53] Hedgal PL, Colvin BA. Potential hazard to Eastern screech owls and other raptors of brodifacoum bait used for vole control in orchards. Environ Toxicol Chem 1988;7:245–60.

[54] Merson MH, Beyers RE, Kaukeinen DE. Residues of the rodenticide brodifacoum in voles and raptors after orchard treatment. J Wildl Manage 1984;48:212–6.

[55] Stone WB, Okoniewski JC, Stedelin JR. Poisoning of wildlife with anticoagulant rodenticides in New York. J Wildl Dis 1999;35:187–93.

[56] Stone WB, Okoniewski JC, Stedelin JR. Anticoagulant rodenticides and raptors: recent findings from New York. Bull Environ Contam Toxicol 2003;70:34–40.

[57] Lassuer R, Grandemange A, Longin-Sauvageon C, et al. Comparison of the inhibition effect of different anticoagulants on vitamin K epoxide reductase activity from warfarin-susceptible and resistant rats. Pestic Biochem Physiol 2007;88(2):203–8.

[58] Warburton PA, Hutson DH. WL 108366-Fate of a single oral dose of 14C-WL 108366 in rats. Part I: Elimination and retention of radioactivity and effect of WL 108366 on prothrombin time. Sittingbourne, Kent: Shell Research Ltd, Sittingbourne Research Centre (Report No. SBGR.85.053); 1985.

[59] United States Environmental Protection Agency, 2006. Memorandum: rodenticide incidents update.

[60] Eason CT, Spurr EB. Review of the toxicity and impacts of brodifacoum on non-target wildlife in New Zealand. N Z J Zool 1995;22:371–9.

[61] Kuijpers EPA, den Hartigh J, Savelkoul TJF, et al. A method for the simultaneous identification and quantitation of five superwarfarin rodenticides in human serum. J Anal Toxicol 1995;19:557–62.

[62] Altman RB, Clubb SL, Dorrestein GM, et al. Avian Medicine and Surgery. Philadelphia: W.B. Saunders; 1997. p. 609.

[63] Ritchie RW, Harrison GJ, Harrison LR. Avian medicine: principles and applications. Lake Worth (FL): Wingers Publishing; 1994. p.1051.

[64] Carpenter JW, Mashima TY, Rupiper DJ. Exotic animal formulary. 2nd edition. Philadelphia: W.B. Saunders; 2001.

[65] LaBonde J. Avian toxicology. Vet Clin North Am Small Anim Pract 1991;21(6):1329–42.

[66] Wells RE, Slocombe RF, Trapp AL. Acute toxicosis in budgerigars (*Melopsittacus undulatus*) caused by pyrolysis products from heated polytetrafluoroethylene: clinical study. Am J Vet Res 1982;43:1238–42.

[67] Forbes NA. PTFE toxicity in birds. Vet Rec 1997;140:512.

VETERINARY
CLINICS
Exotic Animal Practice

Vet Clin Exot Anim 11 (2008) 283–300

Waterfowl Toxicology: A Review

Laurel A. Degernes, DVM, MPH, DABVP–Avian

Department of Clinical Sciences, College of Veterinary Medicine, North Carolina State University, 4700 Hillsborough Street, Raleigh, NC 27606, USA

Free-flying and captive waterfowl are exposed to many potential toxins in their environment, and one should always include toxins on the list of differential diagnoses when investigating a mortality event. This article reviews important anthropogenic (human-related) toxins (lead and other heavy metals, pesticides, and petroleum oil) and natural toxins (botulism, algal toxins, and mycotoxins), including information related to environmental sources, clinical signs, diagnosis, pathologic findings, and treatment options, as applicable.

Heavy metal toxins

Numerous field studies have investigated heavy metal tissue concentrations in free-flying waterfowl, but interpretation of these findings is often challenging. Background and toxic tissue concentrations for different heavy metals in waterfowl vary by species, sex, age, season, geographic region, tissue type, and coaccumulation or interaction with other heavy metals[1]. Some heavy metals are essential as trace nutrients in the diet (eg, zinc, selenium [Se], copper) but may be associated with toxicosis when abnormally elevated levels are present. Most laboratory-based toxicology studies have documented effects of individual heavy metals, often at acutely toxic levels; however, these studies rarely mimic exposures to these elements under field conditions, and few studies have documented interactive effects of concurrent heavy metal exposure (eg, Se may reduce the toxic effects of inorganic and methyl mercury)[1].

Lead toxicosis

Lead toxicosis is one of the most commonly reported toxicities in free-ranging waterfowl. Lead shot was banned nationwide for waterfowl hunting

---

Portions of this article have been adapted from Degernes LA. Toxicities in waterfowl, Semin Avian Exotic Pet Med. 1995;4:15–22, and are used with permission.

E-mail address: laurel_degernes@ncsu.edu

in 1991 and 1997 in the United States and Canada, respectively (Fig. 1). Before these bans, thousands of tons of lead shot were deposited in wetlands and waterfowl habitats. Over time, lead shot sinks to the bottom; is covered by organic and inorganic substrate; and becomes less available to birds foraging for grit or food, such as small mollusks, seeds, or tubers. Spent lead shot ingested by waterfowl is ground in the ventriculus (Figs. 2 and 3) and solubilized by gastric acids before systemic absorption and deposition in soft tissues and bones [2]. Conservative estimates suggest that 1.6 to 2.4 million ducks died annually of lead toxicosis before the ban on lead shot for waterfowl hunting [2]. Since the ban was implemented, studies that compared the prevalence of lead poisoning in waterfowl before and after the ban showed a 44% to 64% reduction in lead poisoning [3,4]. Despite the ban on lead shot use, a vast amount of lead shot remains in the environment and localized problems have continued. Drought conditions in the midwestern states allowed waterfowl to reach previously unattainable spent lead shot in refuges that were closed to hunting for decades [5]. In Washington State, a large number of wild swans died of lead poisoning more than 10 years after lead was banned for waterfowl hunting in that area [6]. Other sources of lead exposure in waterfowl include lead fishing sinkers [6,7], contaminated sediment from mining and smelting operations [8–10], and lead-based paint [11].

The clinical signs of lead toxicosis include weakness, depression, green bile-stained diarrhea, polyuria, anorexia, weight loss, emaciation, subcutaneous edema of the head and eyelids, and behavioral changes [5].

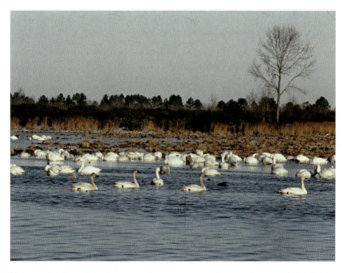

Fig. 1. Wild waterfowl, such as these tundra swans, continue to be at risk for lead toxicosis in some areas in which lead shot was used for waterfowl hunting before the nationwide ban in 1991. (*Courtesy of* L.A. Degernes, DVM, Raleigh, NC.)

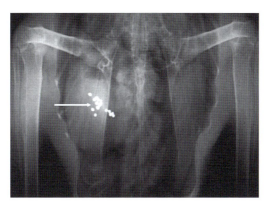

Fig. 2. Toxic (ie, lead) versus nontoxic radiopaque metallic shot pellets (*arrow*) in the ventric-ulus of a waterfowl cannot be differentiated on a radiograph but may be useful for making a preliminary diagnosis of lead toxicosis, pending confirmation of elevated blood lead levels. (*Courtesy of* L.A. Degernes, DVM, Raleigh, NC.)

Neurologic signs range from none to ataxia, tremors, convulsions, drooping wings, partial to complete leg paresis, blindness, or gastrointestinal tract stasis [5,12].

The onset of clinical signs varies with the amount and rate of lead inges-tion and dietary factors. Experimentally poisoned Canada geese given a large number of pellets (n = 25) developed rapid elevations of blood lead concen-tration, acute onset of clinical signs of lead poisoning, and early death within 10 days [13]. Geese dosed with 10 pellets lived longer (up to 72 days), had a slower increase in blood lead concentration, and exhibited signs of chronic lead poisoning. High-fiber diets were associated with more severe

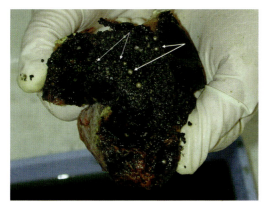

Fig. 3. Shotgun pellets mixed with sand and other grit are present in the ventriculus of a trum-peter swan diagnosed with lead toxicosis. Bold white arrows point toward shiny steel shot, which is more visible than oxidized partially ground-up lead shot, as noted by the narrow white arrows. (*Courtesy of* L.A. Degernes, DVM, Raleigh, NC.)

clinical signs and elevated levels of blood and tissue lead concentration in mallard ducks [14]. Diets higher in natural or supplemented calcium reduced morbidity and mortality in experimentally lead-poisoned ducks [15].

Radiographs (Fig. 2) are useful to detect the presence and quantity of radiopaque metallic pellets in the ventriculus and for identifying birds with an impacted proventriculus [5]. Although nontoxic shot (eg, steel, tungsten matrix, tin, bismuth) and lead cannot be differentiated radiographically, the presence of metallic pellets combined with other supportive evidence is useful in developing a presumptive diagnosis [5]. Some lead-poisoned birds exhibit impaired motility of the ventriculus, as documented with barium fluoroscopy [5].

Hematologic evaluation should include a complete blood cell count, biochemistry profile, and blood lead analysis. Hypochromic regenerative anemia is a consistent finding in lead-poisoned birds [16]. Biochemistry profiles may reflect changes associated with starvation and tissue catabolism but are generally are nondiagnostic for lead toxicosis [17]. Blood lead concentration, measured by atomic absorption spectrophotometry, is useful for establishing a diagnosis and prognosis for lead poisoning [5]. Alternatively, a portable blood lead analyzer may be useful in field studies for rapid identification of birds with elevated lead levels (LeadCare analyzer; ESA, Inc., Chelmsford, Massachusetts) [18]. A blood lead concentration less than 0.5 mg/kg (ppm) is generally not associated with clinical signs and has a good prognosis even without treatment [5]. Blood lead concentrations between 0.5 and 1.0 mg/kg are usually associated with mild to moderate clinical signs and carry a good prognosis for recovery with treatment. The clinical signs and prognosis worsen when blood lead concentrations exceed 1.0 mg/kg. A guarded to poor prognosis is associated with concentrations greater than 2.0 mg/kg.

The delta aminolevulinic acid dehydratase (delta-ALAD) enzyme level is another useful diagnostic test for lead exposure. Lead interferes with red blood cell production by inhibition of two enzymes in the heme synthesis cascade, delta-ALAD and heme synthetase [16]. Inhibition of delta-ALAD enzyme activity (<600 IU/dL) is suggestive of lead exposure or toxicosis.

Private clinical pathology and state diagnostic laboratories have different capabilities and sample requirements for evaluating blood lead and delta-ALAD concentrations in birds. Blood lead concentration is the most useful and readily available diagnostic test for evaluating avian lead toxicosis, but the delta-ALAD enzyme level test is also useful to determine chronicity and prognosis. The reader is encouraged to check with his or her private and state clinical pathology laboratories to determine what services are offered.

The three major components of treatment for lead poisoning include supportive care, chelation, and lead shot removal [5]. Supportive therapy may be required for days to weeks, depending on the degree of debilitation, anemia, and level of lead exposure. Appropriate therapy may include intravenous or intraosseous fluids, tube feeding, and antibiotics and antifungals to treat secondary or concurrent infections. Species that are susceptible to aspergillosis (eg, swans, sea ducks) should be prophylactically treated with itraconazole for the first 7 to 10 days of therapy (5–10 mg/kg administered orally every 24 hours; Sporonox; Janssen Pharmaceutic Products, Titusville, New Jersey) [5,19].

Calcium disodium ethylenediaminetetraacetic acid (CaEDTA) (Versonate; 3M Pharmaceuticals, St. Paul, Minnesota) is a commonly used and effective chelation drug in avian species [5,20]. CaEDTA is administered intravenously (diluted) or intramuscularly at a dosage of 30 to 35 mg/kg twice daily 3 to 5 d/wk for 2 to 6 weeks, depending on the initial blood lead concentration and the presence of metallic lead in the ventriculus [19]. Intramuscular injections are painful and irritating, and intravenous injections are not always possible in smaller avian patients. CaEDTA is also potentially nephrotoxic to the proximal convoluted tubules if used continuously for extended periods [21].

Succimer (Chemet [meso-2,3-dimercaptosuccinic acid (DMSA)]; McNeil-PPC, Inc., Morris Plains, New Jersey) is a relatively safe, water-soluble, heavy metal chelator commonly used for treatment of lead toxicosis in human beings and veterinary patients, including birds [20,22]. Succimer combined with CaEDTA may be more effective than using either drug alone [23]. Succimer was successfully used as an oral chelation agent, with and without CaEDTA therapy, in lead-poisoned trumpeter swans at a dose of 25 to 35 mg/kg administered orally twice daily for 5 d/wk for 3 to 5 weeks [5].

Birds with radiographic evidence of lead pellets or sinkers in the ventriculus are at continued risk for lead toxicosis as long as the metal remains in the ventriculus. Chelation should be continued until all lead is removed from the gastrointestinal tract. Conservative treatments that aid passage of lead include oral administration of mineral oil, magnesium sulfate, high-fiber laxatives, and peanut butter. In the author's experience, these treatments are more effective in psittacines than in waterfowl species. An effective alternative therapy to ventriculotomy is gastric lavage with or without endoscopic retrieval of lead pellets [5]. This procedure is done on an anesthetized intubated bird that is secured to a tilted surgical table with its head and neck pointed down. An appropriately sized flexible stomach tube is passed into the proventriculus, and large quantities of warm water are pumped into the ventriculus using a large syringe. Water pressure and gravity force most of the food, grit, and lead pellets out. Placing a towel over the bucket facilitates collection and analysis of the ventriculus contents and visual examination of the contents for lead pellets. Repeated flushing of water and back-and-forth movement of the stomach tube enhances the flushing action until no more grit washes out. Extreme care should be exercised in birds with proventricular impactions. The proventricular wall may be friable and more susceptible to rupture during gastric lavage therapy. If this approach is unsuccessful in removing all the lead pellets (as determined radiographically), it may be necessary to use an endoscope to remove residual pellets. A flexible endoscope can be used to examine the mucosal lining of the esophagus, proventriculus, and ventriculus for lesions or other problems and to retrieve lead shot [5]. Repeat radiographs of the head, neck, and abdomen should be taken to verify that all the lead has been removed.

Most waterfowl that die of lead poisoning are moderately to severely emaciated, unless they die acutely after a high dose of lead. Nonspecific lesions of lead toxicosis include a bile-distended gallbladder, green liver, bile-stained lining of the ventriculus, and green-stained feathers around the vent [6,24]. Because these changes are also seen with starvation, they are not pathognomonic for lead toxicosis. Impaction of the distal esophagus and proventriculus (Fig. 4) is reported more often in lead-poisoned water-fowl than in other avian species [6,24]. The myocardial muscles (Fig. 5) may be flaccid with grossly visible areas of myocardial degeneration [25]. In geese and swans, cephalic edema and hydropericardium may be present, but these lesions are less common in ducks [12,24].

Histopathologic changes are seen in multiple systems, including renal, gastrointestinal, cardiac, and nervous systems. Hepatic lesions include atro-phy of the hepatocytes, hemosiderin accumulation in the Kupffer cells and hepatocytes, and hepatic necrosis [14]. In birds with proventricular impac-tion, atrophy of the plica and glands in the proventriculus may be present. Renal lesions can include proximal tubular necrosis and degeneration, vis-ceral gout, and acid-fast intranuclear inclusion bodies (not present in every lead-poisoned bird) [13,26]. Myocardial degeneration and necrosis may be secondary to fibrinoid vascular necrosis of arterioles in the heart and other organ locations [13,25]. Fibrinoid vascular necrosis of the duode-num caused severe necrohemorrhagic enteritis in some lead-poisoned swans [5]. Neurologic lesions consist of demyelination of the peripheral nerves, including the vagus, brachial, and sciatic nerves [27]. Experimental lead-induced gonadal lesions in mature roosters showed testicular atrophy and absence of spermatogenesis, but similar lesions have not been reported in waterfowl [28]. Liver lead concentrations greater than 6.0 mg/kg wet weight

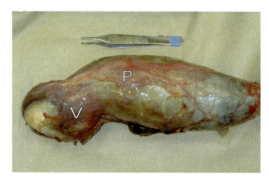

Fig. 4. Food impaction of the proventriculus (P) in a lead-poisoned trumpeter swan resulting in an enlargement three to four times the normal diameter; the ventriculus (V) does not increase in size in lead-poisoned birds. (*Courtesy of* L.A. Degernes, DVM, Raleigh, NC.)

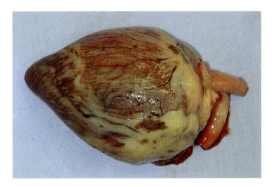

Fig. 5. Pale white streaks of the myocardium in a lead-poisoned trumpeter swan. (*Courtesy of* L.A. Degernes, DVM, Raleigh, NC.)

are generally considered diagnostic, but lower concentrations in context with other significant pathologic changes may also be significant [13,24].

Zinc toxicosis

Zinc toxicosis has been reported in captive and free-flying waterfowl [10,29,30]. Zoologic waterfowl developed zinc toxicosis after ingestion of pennies and fence clips found in their exhibits [29]. US pennies minted after 1983 have approximately 98% zinc. Free-flying waterfowl have also been exposed to toxic levels of zinc in areas contaminated by mining and smelting wastes [10,30]. Nonspecific clinical signs of zinc toxicosis include weakness, ataxia, paresis or paralysis of the legs, anemia, diarrhea, weight loss, and death [10,29,30]. Diagnosis is based on history, clinical signs, radiology, pathologic findings, and elevated serum or tissue (liver, pancreas, or kidneys) zinc concentrations. There is some disagreement with respect to normal versus toxic plasma or serum zinc levels, possibly related to taxonomic differences [31]. General guidelines suggest that plasma or serum zinc levels less than approximately 3 mg/kg are within normal limits and that toxic levels typically exceed 10 mg/kg [29–31]. Interpretation of intermediate zinc levels should include other clinical and diagnostic information to support a diagnosis of zinc toxicosis. The pancreas is the tissue of choice for assessment of zinc toxicosis in birds, but liver and kidney levels are also useful. Mean tissue levels of 530, 440, and 210 mg/kg dry weight were reported in one group of zinc-poisoned waterfowl for the pancreas, liver, and kidneys, respectively [10]. Histopathologic changes include necrotizing ventriculitis and pancreatic necrosis and degeneration [10,29]. A similar therapeutic approach is recommended for zinc toxicosis as is recommended for lead toxicosis; however, if metallic foreign bodies can be removed quickly from the ventriculus, many birds respond favorably to supportive care without the necessity of chelation therapy [29].

Mercury toxicosis

Natural and anthropogenic (human-related) sources of mercury include inorganic and organic (methyl mercury) forms. Documented reports of mercury toxicosis in waterfowl are rare, and most of the information about clinical signs and pathologic findings stem from experimental studies. Methyl mercury is considered the most toxic form for wildlife, especially for the nervous system. This form is readily absorbed, and because it is lipophilic, it easily crosses the blood-brain barrier [32]. Sources of methyl mercury encountered by waterfowl include grains treated with organomercurial fungicides or by means of bioaccumulation of mercury through industrial contamination of aquatic food chains. High concentrations may cause weight loss and weakness in legs and wings, leading to incoordination, the inability to walk or fly, and, ultimately, death [32]. Lower and more chronic exposure is associated with reproduction problems, such as reduced or delayed egg laying, smaller egg size, lowered hatchability, and increased early mortality in ducklings [33]. Background levels of mercury in wild avian liver and kidneys range from 1 to 10 μg/g wet weight, with the higher levels generally associated with scavengers and piscivores [32]. Carnivorous waterfowl, such as mergansers, generally have higher mercury concentrations than herbivorous waterfowl. Presumptive diagnosis of mercury toxicosis is based on kidney tissue residue concentrations exceeding 40 μg/g wet weight [32]. Measurement of concurrent Se levels may be useful for interpretation of elevated mercury levels because Se has been shown to decrease mercury toxicity, even at seemingly toxic levels of mercury [1].

Experimental studies in birds showed that intestinal absorption of inorganic mercury was lower than that of methyl mercury and differed by species. Mallard ducks had lower absorption rates than other birds tested (eg, kestrels, screech owls, bobwhite quail) [32]. Inorganic mercury accumulates predominantly in the kidneys, resulting in proximal renal nephrosis. Other changes include delayed testicular development, gonadal atresia, and decreased fertility of eggs. Treatment has not been reported in waterfowl, but succimer has been successfully used to treat mercury toxicosis in human beings [22].

Cadmium toxicosis

Environmental sources of cadmium (Cd) include industrial and smelting wastes, sewage sludge, burning coal and oils, and phosphate rock fertilizers [34]. Cd bioaccumulates in insects, mollusks, and vertebrates. Cd tissue levels increase with age; however, immature birds may be more susceptible to the toxic effects of Cd than adults [32]. Toxicity studies in adult mallards exposed to Cd at a rate of 200 ppm in their diet for 60 days resulted in mild to severe renal tubular necrosis in many birds and testicular atrophy in 20% of the drakes [35]. In contrast, lower dietary levels of Cd (20 ppm) in mallard ducklings resulted in mild to severe kidney lesions and anemia. Overt Cd toxicity is rarely reported in free-flying waterfowl. Background levels in freshwater ducks are reported to be less than 3 µg/g dry weight in the liver and 2 to 8 µg/g dry weight in the kidneys [36]. Cd levels greater than 40 mg/kg dry weight in the liver or 100 mg/kg dry weight in the kidneys are indicative of toxicosis; however, significant interspecific variation in tissue levels exists in waterfowl [34]. Carnivorous ducks have higher concentrations of Cd than herbivorous or omnivorous waterfowl [36].

Copper toxicosis

Copper toxicosis is rarely reported in free-flying birds; in fact, birds seem to be less susceptible to copper toxicosis compared with fish and aquatic invertebrates [37]. Sources of copper include formulated diets, mining and industrial wastes, pesticides, fungicides, antifouling marine paints, and wood preservatives [37,38]. Toxic tissue concentrations have not been established for waterfowl; however, elevated hepatic copper levels have been reported in free-flying mute swans (*Cygnus olor*) and eiders [38–41]. Hepatic copper levels in seven swans diagnosed with copper poisoning were more than 10 times higher than levels measured in three control swans (mean ± SD: 2150 ± 2280 mg/kg dry weight and 200 ± 140 mg/kg dry weight, respectively) [39]. Hepatic focal necrosis and abundant granules containing copper pigment were observed in these birds [39], and black discolored livers were observed in another group of swans with possible copper toxicosis [38]. There is no known treatment for copper toxicosis.

Selenium toxicosis

Se concentrations are frequently measured in avian field studies, but overt toxicosis is not commonly reported in waterfowl species. Dietary requirements for Se vary by species, and toxic Se concentrations vary by species, age, and interactions with other heavy metals (eg, mercury, zinc, copper), nutrients (eg, vitamin E), and microorganisms [42]. Environmental sources of Se include smelter emissions, sewage sludge, and soils with naturally or artificially elevated levels. One of the most well-documented Se toxicosis problems was in the Kesterson Reservoir in California in the 1980s [43]. Irrigation runoff from agricultural fields naturally high in Se drained into shallow drain water evaporation ponds, in which toxic levels of Se bioaccumulated in plants, invertebrates, and many breeding birds in the area (eg, coots, grebes, shorebirds, ducks) [44]. Adult bird pathologic findings included emaciation, ascites, hepatomegaly, and hepatic necrosis and fibrosis, although gross lesions were not always present [43]. Reduced hatchability and teratogenic abnormalities were observed in many aquatic bird species, including missing or abnormal wings, legs, eyes, or beaks and hydrocephalus [43]. Mean hepatic (94.4 mg/kg dry weight) and renal

(96.6 mg/kg dry weight) Se concentrations measured in American coots (*Fulica americana*) collected at the Kesterson Reservoir were approximately 10 times higher than corresponding levels in control birds [43]. Diagnosis of selenosis can be complicated by its interaction with other metals and nutrients and should include a history of potential exposure, gross and histologic lesions consistent with this toxicosis, or elevated hepatic tissue Se concentration (> 35 mg/kg dry weight) [45]. In laying hens, levels greater than 10 mg/kg may result in reproductive impairment [45].

Pesticide toxicosis

Avian toxicosis has been documented with many pesticide compounds, including organochlorines (OCs), organophosphates (OPs), and carbamates (CAs). OC pesticides, including chlordane, toxaphene, endrin, 1,1, 1-trichloro-2,2-bis(p-chlorophenyl)ethane (DDT) and its analogues, aldrin, dieldrin, and heptachlor, are persistent environmental contaminants. OCs, such as DDT, cause increased firing rates of nerve fibers by decreasing the threshold of the action potential [46]. Acute OC toxicosis has been reported in waterfowl ingesting treated grains or germinating seedlings [47]. Chronic cases of OC toxicosis may develop during periods of malnutrition or stress when stored OC compounds are released after mobilization of fat depots [48]. Clinical signs of OC toxicosis may include muscle fasciculations, spasms and clonic convulsions, ataxia, disorientation, weight loss, and death [46]. The negative effects of OCs on reproductive success have been documented in many avian species, including mallard and black ducks. Egg shell thinning, increased incidence of egg breakage during incubation, and reduced hatchability have been reported in experimental and field exposure studies [48]. These effects persist for more than 2 years after experimental exposure. There are no gross lesions associated with OC toxicosis, except weight loss in chronic cases. Diagnosis is based on elevated concentration of OCs in brain tissue as measured by gas chromatography [48]. There is no known treatment.

OPs (eg, chlorpyrifos, parathion, fenthion, diazinon, dicrotophos, famphur) and CAs (eg, carbofuran, methiocarb, aldcarb) act by inhibiting cholinergic nerve transmission at the neuromuscular junction by inhibiting cholinesterase, which is necessary for hydrolysis of acetylcholine [46]. Acetylcholine accumulation at the neuromuscular junction increases nerve impulse transmission and, ultimately, nerve exhaustion and failure of the nervous system, including respiratory paralysis. Most OPs and CAs are extremely toxic to birds; however, because they are not fat soluble, they do not accumulate in the body and do not persist in the environment. Application of granular formulations of OPs on golf courses and agricultural fields has been associated with acute mortality in waterfowl populations [49,50]. Clinical signs of OP or CA toxicosis associated with overstimulation of the parasympathetic nervous system include diarrhea, excessive salivation and lacrimation, spasm of the nictitans, muscle twitching and tremors, ascending paralysis, and death [51,52].

Diagnosis of OP or CA toxicosis is based on history; clinical signs; and measurement of brain, whole-blood, plasma, or serum cholinesterase concentrations. Although there is considerable species variability regarding OP and CA effects on birds, generally, inhibition of cholinesterase by 20% suggests exposure and greater than 50% inhibition is diagnostic for lethal OP or CA toxicosis [53]. Because cholinesterase activity is reversible with most CA pesticides but not with most OP pesticides, a thermal reactivation technique can be used to differentiate these toxins in brains of pesticide-exposed birds [54]. Brain cholinesterase activity measured before and after 16 to 18 hours of incubation at 36°C to 37°C increases in birds exposed to CA but not to OP compounds. Chemical analysis of crop or proventricular contents may reveal the identity of the pesticide in acute OP toxicosis cases. Lung edema and hyperemia can be observed, but there are usually no gross or histologic lesions with OP or CA toxicosis. The treatment regimen consists of atropine at a dosage of 0.2 mg/kg administered intramuscularly or intravenously, as needed, every 3 to 4 hours until clinical signs resolve [19,55]. When treatment is initiated within 24 hours of exposure, pralidoxime chloride (2-PAM; Protopam; Wyeth-Ayerst Co., Philadelphia, Pennsylvania) at a dose of 10 to 20 mg/kg administered intramuscularly can be used in conjunction with atropine [19].

Botulism

Botulism is caused by ingestion of neuroparalytic toxin (usually type C in waterfowl) produced by the gram-positive anaerobic bacillus *Clostridium botulinum* [56]. Massive die-offs of wild waterfowl populations have been reported, especially in the western United States, and botulism is also a threat to captive waterfowl collections [57].

C botulinum spores are resistant to heat and drying and persist in the environment for long periods. As a result of this persistence, repeated botulism outbreaks in the same area are likely. Environmental conditions that favor botulism outbreaks include warm environmental temperatures, shallow alkaline water that contains abundant invertebrate populations, and decomposing vertebrate carcasses [57]. Waterfowl ingestion of toxin-laden invertebrates or maggots starts the botulism outbreak. The cycle accelerates as more birds die as a result of botulism, more maggots are produced, and more birds ingest the toxic maggots.

Botulism toxin acts by inhibiting release of acetylcholine at the neuromuscular junction, thus preventing impulse transmission [57]. Clinical signs vary with the dose of toxin and time elapsed since ingestion. Early signs of botulism toxicosis include the inability to walk or fly and ataxia, followed by ascending flaccid paralysis of the legs, wings, neck, and nictitating membrane. Death is usually attributable to drowning, respiratory failure, dehydration, or predation.

Birds that die of botulism are generally in good flesh and lack gross or histologic lesions. A presumptive diagnosis is made on the basis of history and clinical signs. Historically, a mouse bioassay test has provided a definitive diagnosis [57]. Two groups of mice are inoculated with test serum, but only one group receives protective antitoxin. Death of unprotected mice and survival of antitoxin-protected mice within 4 to 5 days of inoculation is diagnostic for botulism toxicosis. More recently, ELISA and polymerase chain reaction (PCR) diagnostic tests have also been developed for *C botulism* type C diagnostic testing in wild birds [58,59].

Treatment options for botulism toxicosis depend on the number and types of birds involved. Wild waterfowl with mild signs of botulism can be successfully treated with supportive care, access to fresh water, and shelter from inclement weather and predation [57]. Smaller numbers of birds or more valuable birds from zoos or privately owned collections may benefit from more aggressive fluid and nutritional therapy, administration of type C botulism antitoxin, and gastric lavage to remove toxins and maggots. Prevention of botulism outbreaks in captive waterfowl populations may be difficult in locations with previous outbreaks because of soil contamination. Options include relocation of birds to an uncontaminated site, construction of a deep pond with steep sides, or maintaining stable water levels during the hot summer months to minimize invertebrate die-offs. Constant surveillance for detection and removal of dead birds and other vertebrates is equally important; however, studies have shown that actual detection and removal of carcasses has a low success rate [60]. Mass immunization of wild populations of waterfowl is impractical. A commercial type C toxoid developed for mink (Botumink; United Vaccine, Madison, Wisconsin) provided an insufficient level of protection when administered as a single dose to green-winged teal [61].

Mycotoxicosis

Mycotoxicosis results from ingestion of toxins produced in fungal-contaminated food. Two groups of mycotoxins included in this discussion are aflatoxins and fusariotoxins, which are formed in moldy peanuts or peanut products, corn, and other cereal grains, especially in high-humidity or wet conditions. Diagnosis of mycotoxicosis is difficult and requires identification of the toxin in the food source and demonstration of pathologic lesions. Therefore, most of the literature is based on experimental exposure studies and rarely on field studies. There is no known treatment for these mycotoxins.

Aflatoxins are produced by strains of *Aspergillus* species. Young birds and mallard ducks are more susceptible to aflatoxin B_1 than older birds [62,63]. Acute aflatoxicosis in waterfowl can cause anorexia, depression, ataxia, inability to fly, apparent blindness, and death [62,63]. Liver lesions range from slight hepatomegaly and pale coloration to a slightly shrunken firm liver with a reticulated pattern and ascites. Hepatic necrosis and bile duct hyperplasia are common histologic findings. Aflatoxin exposure may also predispose birds to immunosuppression and hepatic carcinomas [64,65].

Fusariotoxins, such as zearalenone (F2) and tricothecene (T2), are produced from fungi in the genus *Fusarium*. Natural and experimental reports of fusariotoxicosis in waterfowl are uncommon. Clinical signs of T2 toxicosis in waterfowl were nonspecific, including weakness, depression, weight loss, and death [66]. Gross pathologic findings included diphtheritic necrotic lesions in the oral cavity, esophagus, and proventriculus [66,67].

Algal toxicosis

Algal blooms ("red tides") have been associated with acute waterfowl mortality [68]. In one spring outbreak in Florida, a dinoflagellate, *Gymnodinium breve*, was associated with mortality among cormorants, mergansers, and several thousand lesser scaup (*Aythya affinis*) [68]. Clinical signs included weakness, drooping head, flightlessness, oral and nasal discharge, lacrimation, chalky yellow diarrhea, dyspnea, tachypnea, hypothermia, and dehydration. Hematocrits were elevated (50%–70%), gross lesions were absent, and histologic lesions were inconsistent. Toxins produced by another blue-green cyanobacterium, *Anabaena flos-aquae*, have also been documented to cause waterfowl mortality [2]. This toxin causes depolarization at the neuromuscular junction with clinical signs of restlessness, repeated swallowing and salivation, regurgitation, opisthotonos, convulsions, and death. Diagnosis of algal toxicosis can be difficult because signs are nonspecific and it is impossible to detect toxin in the tissue. It is important to collect algal samples and identify the toxins as soon as possible after a suspected outbreak and to rule out other possible causes of mortality, especially botulism. Aquatic birds involved in an outbreak of cyanobacterial toxicosis in Denmark were diagnosed based on stomach contents that were assayed for the presence of algal organisms, tested with microcystin ELISAs, and assayed for anticholinesterase inhibitory activities for anatoxins [69]. Treatment of algal toxicosis is nonspecific, and recommendations include oral administration of activated charcoal and supportive care.

Avian vacuolar myelinopathy (AVM), an emerging neurologic disease linked to cyanobacteria, has caused mortality in bald eagles, American coots, and waterfowl (mallards, ring-necked ducks, buffleheads, and Canada geese) in the southeastern region of the United States since the early 1990s [70–72]. The disease causes microscopic vacuolization of the white matter in the central nervous system (CNS) with clinical signs, such as inability to walk, swim, or fly, and ataxia [73,74]. AVM is generally site specific, seasonal (late fall to early winter), and has a rapid onset of clinical signs after exposure (less than 1 week) [75]. Recent studies have linked a new cyanobacterial species in the order Stigonemetales to AVM, although the specific neurotoxin(s) has not been identified yet [71,72]. Not all birds that have histologic lesions exhibit clinical signs [76], and there are no known treatments for this disease.

Petroleum oil toxicosis

The most common sources of petroleum exposure include oil spills; however, oil pits (waste storage pits and tanks at oil production facilities) have also been associated with avian mortality. One study reported that 10.3% of oiled birds recovered from oil pits were Anseriformes (waterfowl) [77]. Waterfowl exposure to spilled petroleum products can have many deleterious health effects. Destruction of waterproofing and insulation properties of the plumage causes hypothermia [78,79]. Ingestion or inhalation of oil by means of contaminated food, water, or preening may cause pneumonia, diarrhea, hemolytic anemia, and impaired reproduction [78,80–82]. Microliter amounts of oil applied to incubating eggs caused increased embryo mortality [83]. Assessment of marine bird populations (including waterfowl) conducted 9 years after the 1989 Exxon Valdez oil spill in Prince William Sound, Alaska suggested that breeding populations had still not recovered [84]. Magnetic cleansing of oiled feathers using iron powder has been described [85], but most rehabilitation facilities still use a combination of supportive care, antimicrobial agents, and warm water and detergents to treat affected birds [86,87].

References

[1] Goyer RA. Toxic and essential metal interactions. Annu Rev Nutr 1997;17:37–50.
[2] Wobeser GA. Diseases of wild waterfowl. 2nd edition. New York: Plenum Press; 1997. p. 324.
[3] Anderson WL, Havera SP, Zercher BW. Ingestion of lead and nontoxic shotgun pellets by ducks in the Mississippi Flyway. J Wildl Manage 2000;64:848–57.
[4] Samuel MD, Bowers EF. Lead exposure in American black ducks after implementation of non-toxic shot. J Wildl Manage 2000;64:947–53.
[5] Degernes LA, Frank RK, Freeman ML, et al. Lead poisoning in trumpeter swans. Proc Annu Assoc Avian Vet 1989;144–55.
[6] Degernes L, Heilman S, Trogdon M, et al. Epidemiologic investigation of lead poisoning in trumpeter and tundra swans in Washington State, USA, 2000–2002. J Wildl Dis 2006;42:345–58.
[7] Scheuhammer AM, Norris SL. The ecotoxicology of lead shot and lead fishing weights. Ecotoxicology 1996;5:279–95.
[8] Blus LJ, Henny CJ, Hoffman DJ, et al. Lead toxicosis in tundra swans near a mining and smelting complex in northern Idaho. Arch Environ Contam Toxicol 1991;21:549–55.
[9] Sileo L, Creekmore LH, Audet DJ, et al. Lead poisoning of waterfowl by contaminated sediment in the Coeur d'Alene River. Arch Environ Contam Toxicol 2001;41:364–8.
[10] Beyer WN, Dalgarn J, Dudding S, et al. Zinc and lead poisoning in wild birds in the Tri-state Mining District (Oklahoma, Kansas, and Missouri). Arch Environ Contam Toxicol 2005;48: 108–17.
[11] Sileo L, Fefer SI. Paint chip poisoning of Laysan albatross at Midway Atoll. J Wildl Dis 1987;23:432–7.
[12] Bagley GE, Locke LN, Nightingale GT. Lead poisoning in Canada geese in Delaware. Avian Dis 1967;11:601–8.
[13] Cook RS, Trainer DO. Experimental lead poisoning of Canada geese. J Wildl Manage 1966; 30:1–8.

[14] Clemens ET, Krook L, Aronson AL, et al. Pathogenesis of lead shot poisoning in the mallard duck. Cornell Vet 1975;65:248–85.

[15] Carlson BL, Nielsen SW. Influence of dietary calcium on lead poisoning in mallard ducks (*Anas platyrhynchos*). Am J Vet Res 1985;46:276–82.

[16] Lumeij JT. Clinicopathologic aspects of lead poisoning in birds: a review. Vet Q 1985;7:133–8.

[17] March GL, John TM, McKeown BA, et al. The effects of lead poisoning on various plasma constituents in the Canada goose. J Wildl Dis 1976;12:14–9.

[18] Brown CS, Luebbert J, Mulcahy D, et al. Blood lead levels of wild Steller's eiders (*Polysticta stelleri*) and black scoters (*Melanitta nigra*) in Alaska using a portable blood lead analyzer. J Zoo Wildl Med 2006;37:361–5.

[19] Carpenter JW. Exotic animal formulary. 3rd edition. St. Louis (MO): Elsevier Saunders; 2005. p. 592.

[20] Denver MC, Tell LA, Galey FD, et al. Comparison of two heavy metal chelators for treatment of lead toxicosis in cockatiels. Am J Vet Res 2000;61:935–40.

[21] Kowalczyk DF. Clinical management of lead poisoning. J Am Vet Med Assoc 1984;184:858–60.

[22] Graziano JH. Role of 2,3-dimercaptosuccinic acid in the treatment of heavy metal poisoning. Med Toxicol 1986;1:155–62.

[23] Mautino M. Lead and zinc intoxication in zoological medicine: a review. J Zoo Wildl Med 1997;28:28–35.

[24] Beyer WN, Franson JC, Locke LN, et al. Retrospective study of the diagnostic criteria in a lead-poisoning survey of waterfowl. Arch Environ Contam Toxicol 1998;35:506–12.

[25] Karstad L. Angiopathy and cardiopathy in wild waterfowl from ingestion of lead shot. Conn Med 1971;35:355–60.

[26] Simpson VR, Hunt AE, French MC. Chronic lead poisoning in a herd of mute swans. Environ Pollut 1979;18(3):187–202.

[27] Hunter B, Wobeser G. Encephalopathy and peripheral neuropathy in lead-poisoned mallard ducks. Avian Dis 1980;24(1):169–78.

[28] Mazliah J, Barron S, Bental E, et al. The effect of chronic lead intoxication in mature chickens. Avian Dis 1989;33:566–70.

[29] Zdziarski JM, Mattix M, Bush RM, et al. Zinc toxicosis in diving ducks. J Zoo Wildl Med 1994;25:438–45.

[30] Carpenter JW, Andrews GA, Beyer WN. Zinc toxicosis in a free-flying trumpeter swan (*Cygnus buccinator*). J Wildl Dis 2004;40:769–74.

[31] Puschner B, St Leger J, Galey FD. Normal and toxic zinc concentrations in serum/plasma and liver of psittacines with respect to genus differences. J Vet Diagn Invest 1999;11:522–7.

[32] Scheuhammer AM. The chronic toxicity of aluminum, cadmium, mercury, and lead in birds: a review. Environ Pollut 1987;46:263–95.

[33] Heinz G. Effects of low dietary levels of methyl mercury on mallard reproduction. Bull Environ Contam Toxicol 1974;11:386–92.

[34] Furness RW. Cadmium in birds. In: Beyer WN, Heinz GH, Redmon-Norwood AW, editors. Environmental contaminants in wildlife: interpreting tissue concentrations. Clemson University, SC: ETAC Special Publications; 1996. p. 389–404.

[35] White DH, Finley MT, Ferrell JF. Histopathologic effects of dietary cadmium on kidneys and testes of mallard ducks. J Toxicol Environ Health 1978;4:551–8.

[36] Di Giulio RT, Scanlon PF. Heavy metals in tissues of waterfowl from the Chesapeake Bay, USA. Environ Protection (Series A) 1984;35(1):29–48.

[37] Eisler R. Copper hazards to fish, wildlife, and invertebrates: a synoptic review. Washington, DC: US Geological Survey, Biological Resources Division, Biological Science Report; 1998, Contaminant Hazards Review Report No. 33:1–120.

[38] Molnar JJ. Copper storage in the liver of the wild mute swan (*Cygnus olor*): its possible relation to pollution of harbor waters by antifouling paints. Arch Pathol Lab Med 1983;107:629–32.

[39] Kobayashi Y, Shimada A, Umemura T, et al. An outbreak of copper poisoning in mute swans (*Cygnus olor*). J Vet Med Sci 1992;54:229–33.

[40] Elvestad K, Karlog O, Clausen B. Heavy metals (copper, cadmium, lead, mercury) in mute swans from Denmark. Nord Vet Med 1982;34:92–7.

[41] Stout JH, Trust KA, Cochrane JF, et al. Environmental contaminants in four eider species from Alaska and Arctic Russia. Environ Pollut 2002;119:215–26.

[42] Eisler R. Selenium hazards to fish, wildlife, and invertebrates: a synoptic review. Washington, DC: US Fish and Wildlife Service Biological Report; 1985, Contaminant Hazards Reviews Report No. 5:1–41.

[43] Ohlendorf HM, Kilness AW, Simmons JL, et al. Selenium toxicosis in wild aquatic birds. J Toxicol Environ Health 1988;24:67–92.

[44] Ohlendorf HM, Hothem RL, Bunck CM, et al. Bioaccumulation of selenium in birds at Kesterson Reservoir, California. Arch Environ Contam Toxicol 1990;19:495–507.

[45] Heinz GH. Selenium in birds. In: Beyer WN, Heinz GH, Redmon-Norwood AW, editors. Environmental contaminants in wildlife: interpreting tissue concentrations. Clemson University (SC): ETAC Special Publications; 1996. p. 447–58.

[46] Walker CH. Neurotoxic pesticides and behavioural effects upon birds. Ecotoxicology 2003; 12:307–16.

[47] Stanley PI, Bunyan PJ. Hazards to wintering geese and other wildlife from the use of dieldrin, chlorfenvinphos and carbophenothion as wheat seed treatments. Proc R Soc Lond B Biol Sci 1979;205:31–45.

[48] Blus LJ. DDT, DDD, and DDE in birds. In: Beyer WN, Heinz GH, Redmon-Norwood AW, editors. Environmental contaminants in wildlife: interpreting tissue concentrations. Clemson University, SC: ETAC Special Publications; 1996. p. 49–71.

[49] Kendall RJ, Brewer LW, Hitchcock RR, et al. American wigeon mortality associated with turf application of diazinon AG500. J Wildl Dis 1992;28:263–7.

[50] White DH, Mitchell CA, Kolbe EJ, et al. Parathion poisoning of wild geese in Texas. J Wildl Dis 1982;18:389–91.

[51] Odenkirchen EW, Eisler R. Chlorpyrifos hazards to fish, wildlife, and invertebrates: a synoptic review. Washington, DC: US Fish and Wildlife Service Biological Report; 1988, Contaminant Hazard Reviews Report No. 13:1–24.

[52] Eisler R. Carbofuran hazards to fish, wildlife, and invertebrates: a synoptic review. Washington, DC: US Fish and Wildlife Service Biological Report; 1985, Contaminant Hazard Reviews Report No. 3:1–23.

[53] Melancon MJ, et al. Bioindicators used in aquatic and terrestrial monitoring. In: Hoffman DJ, Rattner BA, Burton GA, editors. Handbook of ecotoxicology. Boca Raton (FL): Lewis Publishers, CRC Press, Inc; 1995. p. 220–30.

[54] Smith MR, Thomas NJ, Hulse C. Application of brain cholinesterase reactivation to differentiate between organophosphorus and carbamate pesticide exposure in wild birds. J Wildl Dis 1995;31:263–7.

[55] LaBonde J. Avian toxicology. Vet Clin North Am Small Anim Pract 1991;21:1329–42.

[56] Wobeser G. Avian botulism—another perspective. J Wildl Dis 1997;33:181–6.

[57] Locke LN, Friend M. Avian botulism. In: Davidson WR, Nettles VF, editors. Field manual of wildlife diseases in the southeastern United States. University of Georgia, Athens, GA: Southeastern Cooperative Wildlife Disease Study; 1988. p. 83–93.

[58] Rocke TE, Smith SR, Nashold SW. Preliminary evaluation of a simple *in vitro* test for the diagnosis of type C botulism in wild birds. J Wildl Dis 1998;34:744–51.

[59] Franciosa G, Fenicia L, Caldiani C, et al. PCR for detection of *Clostridium botulinum* type C in avian and environmental samples. J Clin Microbiol 1996;34:882–5.

[60] Cliplef DJ, Wobeser G. Observations on waterfowl carcasses during a botulism epizootic. J Wildl Dis 1993;29:8–14.

[61] Rocke TE, Samuel MD, Swift PK, et al. Efficacy of a type C botulism vaccine in green-winged teal. J Wildl Dis 2000;36:489–93.

[62] Robinson RM, Ray AC, Reagor JC, et al. Waterfowl mortality caused by aflatoxicosis in Texas. J Wildl Dis 1982;18:311–3.

[63] Muller RD, Carlson CW, Semeniuk G, et al. The response of chicks, ducklings, goslings, pheasants and poults to graded levels of aflatoxins. Poult Sci 1970;49:1346–50.

[64] Cullen JM, Marion PL, Sherman GJ, et al. Hepatic neoplasms in aflatoxin B1-treated, congenital duck hepatitis B virus-infected, and virus-free Pekin ducks. Cancer Res 1990; 50:4072–80.

[65] Hurley DJ, Neiger RD, Higgins KF, et al. Short-term exposure to subacute doses of aflatoxin-induced depressed mitogen responses in young mallard ducks. Avian Dis 1999; 43:649–55.

[66] Hayes MA, Wobeser GA. Subacute toxic effects of dietary T-2 toxin in young mallard ducks. Can J Comp Med 1983;47:180–7.

[67] Shlosberg AS, Klinger Y, Malkinson MH. Muscovy ducklings, a particularly sensitive avian bioassay for T-2 toxin and diacetoxyscirpenol. Avian Dis 1986;30:820–4.

[68] Forrester DJ, Gaskin JM, White FH, et al. An epizootic of waterfowl associated with a red tide episode in Florida. J Wildl Dis 1977;13:160–7.

[69] Henriksen P, Carmichael WW, An J, et al. Detection of an anatoxin-a(s)-like anticholinesterase in natural blooms and cultures of cyanobacteria/blue-green algae from Danish lakes and in the stomach contents of poisoned birds. Toxicon 1997;35:901–13.

[70] Fischer JR, Lewis-Weis LA, Tate CM, et al. Avian vacuolar myelinopathy outbreaks at a southeastern reservoir. J Wildl Dis 2006;42:501–10.

[71] Wilde SB, Murphy TM, Hope CP, et al. Avian vacuolar myelinopathy linked to exotic aquatic plants and a novel cyanobacterial species. Environ Toxicol 2005;20:348–53.

[72] Wiley FE, Wilde SB, Birrenkott AH, et al. Investigation of the link between avian vacuolar myelinopathy and a novel species of cyanobacteria through laboratory feeding trials. J Wildl Dis 2007;43:337–44.

[73] Thomas NJ, Meteyer CU, Sileo L. Epizootic vacuolar myelinopathy of the central nervous system of bald eagles (*Haliaeetus leucocephalus*) and American coots (*Fulica americana*). Vet Pathol 1998;35:479–87.

[74] Larsen RS, Nutter FB, Augspurger T, et al. Clinical features of avian vacuolar myelinopathy in American coots. J Am Vet Med Assoc 2002;221:80–5.

[75] Rocke TE, Thomas NJ, Augspurger T, et al. Epizootiologic studies of avian vacuolar myelinopathy in waterbirds. J Wildl Dis 2002;38:678–84.

[76] Fischer JR, Lewis-Weis LA, Tate CM. Experimental vacuolar myelinopathy in red-tailed hawks. J Wildl Dis 2003;39:400–6.

[77] Trail PW. Avian mortality at oil pits in the United States: a review of the problem and efforts for its solution. Environ Manage 2006;38:532–44.

[78] Balseiro A, Espi A, Marquez I, et al. Pathological features in marine birds affected by the Prestige's oil spill in the north of Spain. J Wildl Dis 2005;41:371–8.

[79] Jenssen BM. Effects of ingested crude and dispersed crude oil on thermoregulation in ducks (*Anas platyrhynchos*). Environ Res 1989;48:49–56.

[80] Leighton FA. Clinical, gross, and histological findings in herring gulls and Atlantic puffins that ingested Prudhoe Bay crude oil. Vet Pathol 1986;23:254–63.

[81] Leighton FA, Peakall DB, Butler RG. Heinz-body hemolytic anemia from the ingestion of crude oil: a primary toxic effect in marine birds. Science 1983;220:871–3.

[82] Harvey S, Klandorf H, Phillips JG. Reproductive performance and endocrine responses to ingested petroleum in domestic ducks (*Anas platyrhynchos*). Gen Comp Endocrinol 1981;45: 372–80.

[83] Couillard CM, Leighton FA. Comparative pathology of Prudhoe Bay crude oil and inert shell sealants in chicken embryos. Fundam Appl Toxicol 1989;13:165–73.

[84] Lance BK, Irons DB, Kendall SJ, et al. An evaluation of marine bird population trends following the Exxon Valdez oil spill, Prince William Sound, Alaska. Mar Pollut Bull 2001; 42:298–309.

[85] Orbell JD, Ngeh LN, Bigger SW, et al. Whole-bird models for the magnetic cleansing of oiled feathers. Mar Pollut Bull 2004;48:336–40.
[86] Lauer DM, Frink J, Dein FJ. Rehabilitation of ruddy ducks contaminated with oil. J Am Vet Med Assoc 1982;181:1398–9.
[87] Jenssen BM. Review article: effects of oil pollution, chemically treated oil, and cleaning on thermal balance of birds. Environ Pollut 1994;86:207–15.

ELSEVIER
SAUNDERS

VETERINARY
CLINICS
Exotic Animal Practice

Vet Clin Exot Anim 11 (2008) 301–314

Toxicology of Ferrets

Eric Dunayer, MS, VMD, DABT, DABVT[a,b],*

[a]*American Society for the Prevention of Cruelty to Animals (ASPCA) Animal Poison Control Center (APCC), 1717 S. Philo Road, Suite 36, Urbana, IL 61802, USA*
[b]*College of Veterinary Medicine, University of Illinois, 2001 S. Lincoln Avenue, Urbana, IL 61802, USA*

Ferrets are prone to toxicoses for several reasons. First, they are curious by nature, leading them to explore areas where potential toxicants exist. Second, their strong jaws and sharp teeth allow them to open pill vials and sealed containers [1]. Finally, because of their small size (generally less than 2 kg [2]), even small ingestions of a toxicant can lead to a large dosage on a mg/kg basis.

One important note: The literature on ferret toxicosis is sparse and much of the information in this article is based on information from dogs and cats. More up-to-date information for a particular toxicosis in ferrets may be available by calling the American Society for the Prevention of Cruelty to Animals (ASPCA) Animal Poison Control Center (APCC) at 1-888-426-4435. In most cases, this is a fee-based service.

Initial considerations

One of the basics tenets of toxicology is "Treat the patient, not the poison"[3]. Therefore, the initial approach to poisoning in a ferret is no different from any other species. On presentation, the patient (particularly if symptomatic) should be evaluated and stabilized, including control of arrhythmias, respiratory distress, seizures, and so forth [3]. Only then should a thorough history and complete physical be performed. Physical examination and common procedures that may be appropriate to a poisoned ferret have been discussed elsewhere [4].

The likelihood of a toxicosis causing the ferret's signs should be determined. Many people believe that the sudden onset of signs in an apparently

---

* ASPCA, Animal Poison Control Center, 1717 S. Philo Road, Suite 36, Urbana, IL 61802.

E-mail address: ericdunayer@aspca.org

1094-9194/08/$ - see front matter © 2008 Elsevier Inc. All rights reserved.
doi:10.1016/j.cvex.2008.01.001   *vetexotic.theclinics.com*

302   DUNAYER

healthy animal is most likely due to a toxicosis. The clinician should determine whether the exposure was witnessed, whether strong evidence of an exposure exists (eg, a chewed-open pill container with missing medication), or
the owner only suspects an intoxication because of sudden onset of signs. In
cases where the exposure is not certain, the clinician should pursue a thorough work-up to determine other causes of the signs [3]. If possible, blood
should be drawn before any medications are given to avoid possible interference with clinical laboratory tests. History should include questions about
the environment, whether the animal was unsupervised, what toxicants
are in the environment, behavior changes before the onset of the signs,
and so forth [3].

Decontamination

Early decontamination may be useful in preventing or limiting signs that
can develop from a toxic exposure. The decision whether or not to decon-
taminate the patient should be based on the risk associated from the exposure as well as the patient's current condition. Procedures such as inducing
emesis or administering activated charcoal do carry risks for the patient. In
some instances, especially when the exposure is unlikely to cause significant
signs, no treatment may be indicated.

Since ferrets can vomit, emesis may be attempted depending on the exposure [1]. For instance, emesis should not be induced for corrosives such as
alkalis, acids, and cationic detergents, because emesis can reexpose the
esophagus and oral cavity to the corrosive materials [1]. Inducing emesis
after ingestion of petroleum distillates increases the risk of aspiration.
Finally, if the animal is already symptomatic—vomiting, depressed, seizuring, and so forth—emesis should not be attempted [3].

Emesis can be achieved with the use of 3% hydrogen peroxide [1]. In general, results are improved if there is food present in the stomach [1]. If the
ferret has not eaten recently, a small meal should be fed before inducing
emesis. Because hydrogen peroxide tends to lose its potency over time, the
solution should be checked before usage for activity by pouring a small
amount of the hydrogen peroxide into a sink and observing for bubbling
or foaming. The dose of hydrogen peroxide is 1 mL/lb (0.45 mL/kg) [1].
After administering hydrogen peroxide, the ferret should be encouraged
to be active to increase "agitation" of the hydrogen peroxide [3]. Most
animals should vomit within 10 to 15 minutes. If the initial dose is not
successful, one additional dose of hydrogen peroxide can be administered.
After emesis, the mouth can be rinsed to remove any remaining hydrogen
peroxide [1]. Be sure that the ferret is not allowed to re-ingest the vomitus.

Syrup of ipecac can be used; however, it takes longer to work than hydrogen peroxide and there is a risk of cardiac toxicity if emesis does not occur.
Syrup of ipecac is being taken off the market so it is unlikely it will be
available in the future. One study found that vomiting in ferrets occurred

at doses of 0.25 to 1 mL/kg [5]. Other agents such as diluted liquid dishwashing detergent or dried mustard can be used in an emergency situation if nothing else is available [3]; however, they are unreliable. Salt should never be used as an emetic because it can cause life-threatening hypernatremia especially if the animal does not vomit [3].

At the veterinary clinic, emesis can be induced using apomorphine. It can be administered at 0.04 mg/kg intravenously (IV), subcutaneously (SQ), or intramuscularly (IM). Alternatively, the apomorphine can be dissolved in sterile water or saline and placed in the conjunctival sac at a dose of 0.25 mg/kg [3]. Following emesis, the eye can be flushed to remove any remaining drug. The patient should be monitored for signs of excessive sedation or agitation. These signs can be reversed with a standard dose of naloxone [3].

Gastric lavage can be useful in some instances but may be of limited value in the ferret. First, the animal must be anesthetized and a cuffed endrotracheal tube placed to avoid aspiration [3]. Second, because of their small size, the diameter of the stomach tube that can be passed may severely limit the amount of material that can be recovered, especially if the agent does not dissolve easily. Finally, gastric lavage should not be used for caustics and petroleum distillates [1]. Lavage fluid should be instilled and recovered by gravity; the lavage should be continued until the fluid runs clear [3].

If there may be a large amount of unabsorbed material in the intestines, an enterogastric lavage can be performed. In this procedure, a gastric lavage is performed first. Then, a tube is passed rectally and a high enema under low water pressure is performed to propel intestinal material cranially. The enema is continued until enema fluid passes through the gastric tube and finally runs clear [3].

For ingestion of caustics—in which emesis is contraindicated—dilution is the initial treatment of choice [1]. Milk, yogurt, or water can be given orally to dilute the caustic and reduce the damage it may do. Small volumes (0.25 to 0.50 teaspoon) should be used to avoid causing spontaneous emesis [3].

After emesis, or possibly instead of emesis, activated charcoal should be administered if indicated. Substances such as caustics, petroleum distillates, and metals are poorly absorbed by activated charcoal and so its use is not recommended in such exposure. Similarly, small molecules like ethanol and ethylene glycol are also poorly absorbed [3]. The dose of activated charcoal is 1 to 3 g/kg [1]. For agents that undergo enterohepatic recirculation or are extended release formulations, multiple doses of activated charcoal every 6 to 8 hours may be useful [3]. When multiple doses are used, half the original dose should be administered for the additional doses [3]. Because many activated-charcoal preparations contain osmotically active ingredients, a shift of free water into the gut can occur with a secondary hypernatremia resulting. The ferret should be watched for about 4 hours after the activated charcoal is administered for signs of hypernatremia such as ataxia, tremors, or seizures. Acute hypernatremia can be treated by rapidly lowering the serum sodium with low-sodium intravenous fluids such as 5% dextrose in water or $\frac{1}{2}$ str. saline and dextrose. Additionally, plain-water enemas (5 to 10 mL/kg) can be given to take advantage of the colon's ability to absorb water rapidly [3].

A cathartic (often premixed in with the activated charcoal) can also be administered to decrease transport time through the gut. Common cathartics include sorbitol, magnesium sulfate, and bulk laxatives [1]. Because of the risk of dehydration and hypernatremia, cathartics should not be administered more than once a day if multiple doses of activated charcoal are being given.

For exposure to topical toxicants, the ferret's coat and skin should be thoroughly rinsed; a mild shampoo may also be used [1]. Many agents, such as spot-on flea products, tend to be oily and may not be easily removed by just plain water. In these instances, a bath with a liquid dishwashing detergent (such as Dawn) can be performed to remove the agent [1]. The patient should be kept warm after the bath. For animals showing neurologic signs, baths should be delayed until the signs have been adequately controlled as the stress of bathing may exacerbate the signs.

For ocular exposure, the eye should be flushed for 20 to 30 minutes total. Saline is the preferred agent. However, if saline is not available, distilled or tepid tap water can be used. Medicated eye drops or disinfecting contact lens solutions should not be used. After flushing, fluorescein stain can be used to determine if a corneal ulcer is present [3].

Specific agents

Between November 2001 and September 2007, the APCC handled 618 cases of ferrets suspected or observed exposure to various toxicants (ASPCA APCC unpublished data, 2007). Box 1 shows the most common exposures reported to the APCC. Most of the exposures (over 50% of reported cases) occurred to various medications with only a few cases for each medication. To discuss every agent that a ferret could be exposed to is well beyond this article's scope, but the more common exposures will be discussed.

Cleaning products (including bleaches)

Most cleaning agents consist of anionic/nonionic surfactants. These agents are irritants but significant systemic toxicity is not expected [6]. Small ingestions may lead to nausea and vomiting. Large ingestions may also cause diarrhea due to a laxative effect. Immediate treatment consists of diluting the agent with milk or water to reduce irritation. Vomiting can usually be managed symptomatically by withholding food and water for a few hours. In more severe cases, correction of dehydration, electrolyte imbalances, and vomiting may be needed [6].

Bleach and other alkaline corrosive products can cause tissue damage ranging from irritation to corrosion. The degree of injury depends on

---

Box 1. Most common exposure reported to the APCC

Miscellaneous medications
Cleaning products (including bleaches)
Insecticides
Flea products
Ibuprofen
Anticoagulant rodenticides
Chocolate
Acetaminophen
Venlafaxine (Effexor)
Bromethalin
Toxic plants
Paint
Soaps and shampoos

From November 2001 to September 2007 (10 or more reports of 618 cases).

---

concentration of the corrosive. While dilute solutions may be irritating, concentrated solutions may be extremely alkaline and those with a pH greater than 11 are corrosive [7]. Because pain is not immediate, animals may continue to consume large amounts of the agent [8]. Therefore, the injury may extend beyond the oral cavity and include damage to the esophagus and stomach. In addition, the full extent of the injury may not be evident for 24 hours. Immediate care for alkaline corrosive ingestion is dilution with milk or water. Emesis is contraindicated. Activated charcoal does not bind these agents and may impede healing of ulcers. Attempts to neutralize an alkaline substance with an acid are contraindicated as this may lead to the release of heat, which can further damage soft tissue [8]. The patient should be monitored for at least 24 hours [7]. Soft food should be fed to reduce irritation to any damaged tissue. If ulcers or burns should develop, liquid or slurried carafate should be given (75 mg/kg by mouth every 4 to 6 hours) [9] to protect ulcers while healing. Antibiotics may be necessary. Nutritional support, including feeding tubes, is indicated if the ferret is not eating [7]. The animal should also be monitored for signs of esophageal stricture/perforation for 2 to 3 weeks [8]. Steroids have been suggested for use in reducing esophageal scarring; however, their use is considered controversial as they increase the risk of infection [8]. Dermal and ocular exposures are treated as outlined in the decontamination section.

Insecticides

Ferrets may be exposed to insecticides through a variety of products including sprays, granules, dusts, and baits. Most insecticidal products currently contain ingredients with lower toxicity. These agents include pyre-throids [10], fipronil [11], hydramethylnon [11], and sulfluramid [11]. These ingredients have a wide margin of safety and generally are present in low concentrations in the products. In general, they may cause mild to moderate gastrointestinal upset if ingested (often because of the inert ingredients in the formulation) but severe systemic signs are rarely seen. The treatment is symptomatic and supportive.

Topical flea products

When used according to label, topical flea products are generally of very low toxicity [12]. Any topically applied agent may cause dermal irritation or a hypersensitivity reaction. However, problems may arise when a product is used on a species for which it is not labeled. For instance, cats may develop tremors or seizures following application of concentrated (45% to 65%) per-methrin spot-on products labeled for dogs [10], while dermal application of fipronil in rabbits may lead to seizures [11]. Similar claims have been made for pyrethrin- and pyrethroids-products and ferrets [13,14]. On the other hand, one article reported that when a 50% permethrin with 10% imidaclor-prid spot-on was used on farmed mink (*Mustela vison*), the agent was found to be effective and there was no mention of toxicity in the animals [15]. However, signs can be seen in an overdose situation such as when the entire contents of a tube of permethrin spot-on labeled for large dogs is applied to a ferret. In any case, because the use of these products is off-label, veterinar-ians should encourage their clients to use only those products approved for use in ferrets.

If a flea product is used off-label on a ferret, the best advice is to prevent further exposure to that product though dermal decontamination. A bath using a liquid hand-dishwashing product (such as Dawn) should be per-formed and the ferret kept warm [10]. Since these agents tend to be lipo-philic, regular pet shampoos may not be strong enough to remove the insecticide. In symptomatic ferrets, bathing should be delayed until the neu-rologic signs are controlled; otherwise, the stress of bathing may worsen the signs. In addition, the animal should be kept warm following the bath, as hypothermia may worsen tremors especially with pyrethroids [10].

In animals that are tremoring because of pyrethroid toxicosis, methocar-bamol is the treatment of choice [10]. (Diazepam usually does not control the tremors associated with permethrin [10]). The recommended dose is 55 to 220 mg/kg slow IV. The methocarbamol should be administered in 55-mg/kg boluses until the worst of the tremors are controlled. Generally, a 330-mg/kg/day dosage should not be exceeded [10]. Oral methocarbamol can be used if the injectable form is not available; it can be dissolved in saline and given rectally. If methocarbamol is not effective, barbiturates may be used but the animal must be watched closely for respiratory depres-sion. For seizures, diazepam may be effective [10].

The use of alcohol-based flea sprays may predispose the ferret to alcohol toxicity. The author has seen several cases in which animals were soaked with an alcohol-based product then confined to a small area such as a carrier. Later the animals were found to be severely ataxic or moribund. Alcohols can be absorbed dermally as well as inhaled. Signs include ataxia, hypothermia, hypoglycemia, acidosis, and coma. Treatment is supportive and symptomatic and includes rinsing the product off, IV fluids ± dextrose, thermoregulation, and respiratory support if needed [16].

Ibuprofen

Ibuprofen is a common nonsteroidal anti-inflammatory drug (NSAID) used for the control of pain. It is available in several different forms. Over-the-counter forms include 50-, 100-, and 200-mg tablets and as well as 20-mg/mL and 40-mg/mL liquids for children. Prescription strength includes 400-, 600-, and 800-mg tablets [17]. Ibuprofen inhibits the production of prostaglandins associated with pain. However, especially in an overdose situation, it can also inhibit prostaglandins that protect the gastric mucosa, predisposing the animal to gastric ulcers and those that maintain normal renal-blood flow, which can lead to acute renal failure [18].

A review of ibuprofen ingestion by ferrets at the APCC [19] showed that signs developed within 4 hours in about 40% of the ferrets, with the rest developing signs up to 48 hours postexposure. Neurologic signs were the most common signs seen in about 95% of the ferrets; signs included depression, coma, ataxia, and tremors. Neurologic signs can be seen in dogs ingesting ibuprofen but generally require a much larger dose than seen in this study [18]. Slightly more than half the ferrets also showed gastrointestinal signs including anorexia, vomiting and retching, diarrhea, and melena. Renal signs including polyuria, polydipsia, and renal failure may also be seen. The minimum lethal dose was 220 mg/kg [18]; in a small ferret this could be a single 200-mg ibuprofen tablet.

If the ingestion is discovered before signs have occurred, standard decontamination procedures (emesis and/or activated charcoal) can be performed. Because ibuprofen undergoes enterohepatic recirculation, multiple doses of activated charcoal may be useful [18].

However, if the ferret presents comatose, decontamination should be delayed until the animal is stabilized. Treatment may include IV fluids, oxygen, and thermoregulation. Gastric lavage may be performed but an endrotracheal tube must be placed to prevent aspiration. Activated charcoal can be left in the stomach after the lavage is performed. Various gastrointestinal protectants should be started; Table 1 shows suggested doses. An acid-reducer such as famotidine combined with carafate should be administered for 5 to 7 days; longer if the animal continues to show signs [19]. Misoprostol, a synthetic prostaglandin, can also be used for the first 48 hours; however, since it comes in 100-μg tablets, it may be difficult to dose the

Table 1
Suggested drugs and dosages for treating ibuprofen toxicity in ferrets [18]

Drug	Recommended dosages
Acid Reducers	
Cimetidine	5–10 mg/kg PO, SQ, IM, IV q8 h
Famotidine	0.25–0.5 mg/kg PO, IV q24 h
Sucralfate	0.125 g q6 h PO
Misoprostol	1–5 µg/kg PO q8 h
Metoclopromide	0.2–1 mg/kg PO, SQ

Abbreviations: IM, intramuscular; IV, intravenous; PO, by mouth; q, every; SQ, subcutaneous.

ferret unless the agent is compounded to a more usable concentration. Finally, vomiting can be controlled using metoclopromide or similar anti-emetic. Baseline BUN (blood urea nitrogen), creatinine, and phosphorus should be determined. Fluid diuresis at twice the maintenance rate for 48 hours should be performed to maintain renal blood flow and reduce the risk of acute renal failure [19].

With early decontamination and treatment, the prognosis for ibuprofen ingestion in ferrets is good. However, once symptoms occur, especially if the ferret is comatose or seizuring, the prognosis is guarded to grave.

Anticoagulant rodenticides

Anticoagulant rodenticides include compounds such as warfarin and so-called second-generation agents such as bromadiolone, chlorophacinone, diaphacinone, brodifacoum, and difethialone [20]. These agents interfere with the liver's production of clotting factors II, VI, IX, and X. Following depletion of these factors hemorrhage may begin, generally 3 to 7 days after ingestion of the agent. Initial signs may be vague and include lethargy and inappetance. Signs of hemorrhage may not be evident until late in the toxicosis. Bleeding may occur into the chest, abdomen, under the skin, and/or in the central nervous system (CNS) [20].

These agents are extremely potent. Because of lack of toxicologic data in ferrets and the great variation of toxic doses in the literature, the APCC uses 0.02 mg/kg as a dosage at which decontamination and treatment should be performed [20]. For the average ferret, this would be about 0.5 to 1.0 g of a 0.005% bait (the most common concentration).

For ingestions of less than 4 hours, emesis can be performed. In addition, activated charcoal may be of benefit. Because of the narrow margin of safety for these agents, vitamin K1 should be started at a dose of 5 mg/kg divided every 8 to 12 hours [21]. Injection of vitamin K1 should be avoided as both IV and SQ injections can cause anaphylactic reactions [20,21]. Because of their small size, it may be difficult to dose ferrets with oral vitamin K1 preparations (which generally come as 5-, 25-, or 50-mg tablets). Instead, inject-able vitamin K1 can be given orally [21] or an appropriate solution can be compounded [20]. It is important that vitamin K1 be given with a fatty food (such as peanut butter or canned cat food), as bile acids are needed for proper absorption [20,21]. The course of treatment depends on the agent. After warfarin ingestion, vitamin K1 should be given for at least 2 weeks, bromadiolone requires a minimum of 3 weeks of treatment, while all other second-generation anticoagulant rodenticides should be treated for at least 28 days [21]. Forty-eight hours after stopping vitamin K1, a prothrombin time (PT) should be performed to determine if the treatment has been successful. If the PT is elevated, an additional week of vitamin K1 should be prescribed and the PT rechecked again after stopping the medication. Normal values for ferrets may not be available [21] in which case a second sample from a normal ferret may need to be assayed to interpret the results.

In ferrets that present symptomatic, treatment should be aimed at stopping hemorrhage, correcting anemia if present, and starting vitamin K1. Because there is a 24- to 48-hour lag period before the liver starts to produce adequate levels of clotting factors, plasma can provide clotting factors for stopping hemorrhage. If plasma is not available, blood can be drawn from a donor ferret and the plasma separated by allowing the red blood cells (RBCs) to settle or by centrifuging anticoagulated blood in sterile tubes. Fresh whole blood can be used but the clinician should monitor the patient closely for volume overload, particularly if the patient is not anemic [20]. Vitamin K1, as outlined above, should be started.

Chocolate

Because it is sweet and contains a high percentage of fat, chocolate may be a tempting treat for ferrets. Chocolate, however, contains methylxanthines (principally theobromine and caffeine), which are cardiac and CNS stimulants [8]. Table 2 contains the relative amounts of methylxanthines found in the most common forms of chocolates. In generally, total methylxanthine dosages around 10 to 15 mg/kg result in gastrointestinal upset (principally vomiting and diarrhea). At dosages greater than 40 to 50 mg/kg, tachycardia can be seen, while dosages greater than 60 mg/kg can result in CNS stimulation with tremors and seizures, and doses over 100 mg/kg may be acutely fatal [8].

Treatment for chocolate intoxication is supportive and symptomatic. Since chocolate tends to stay in the stomach for a long period after ingestion,

Table 2
Representative theobromine and caffeine content of various chocolates

Compound	Theobromine, mg/oz	Caffeine, mg/oz
White chocolate	0.25	0.85
Milk chocolate	44–56	6
Semi-sweet chocolate chips	138	22
Baker's chocolate (unsweetened)	393	8–18
Dry cocoa powder	130–737	5–42

Based on information collected by the Animal Poison Control Center.

emesis may be useful for up to 8 hours following ingestion. Activated charcoal should be administered as well; multiple doses may be useful and should be administered every 6 to 8 hours as long as the ferret is symptomatic. Fluid diuresis will help with excretion of methylxanthines so intravenous fluids at twice-maintenance levels should be started. Because caffeine can be reabsorbed through the bladder wall, the ferret should be encouraged to void. If the animal is not able to urinate, a urinary catheter can be placed [8].

In symptomatic animals, treatment is aimed at controlling the signs. Tachycardia can be controlled by beta-blockers such as propranolol. CNS stimulation and seizures should respond to diazepam. Spontaneous vomiting can be handled by an appropriate antiemetic [8].

Acetaminophen

Acetaminophen is a pain reliever commonly taken for control of fever, headaches, and joint or muscle pain [22]. It is often combined with other medications, especially opioids [23]. Overdoses of acetaminophen in ferrets can lead to acute hepatic necrosis, methemoglobinemia, and, rarely, acute renal failure [22,23]. Ferret RBCs appear to be especially sensitive to oxidative stress and so may be prone to formation of methemoglobinemia with exposure to acetaminophen [13]. In one study [24], ferrets were dosed at 50, 100, or 200 mg/kg with acetaminophen. Lethargy and anorexia occurred in most ferrets in the study regardless of dose and half the ferrets in the 200-mg/kg dosage group died. However, the study did not report on clinical pathologic changes in the ferrets.

Standard decontamination (emesis and/or activated charcoal) should be performed early in the toxicosis. A minimum baseline blood panel including liver enzymes (alanine aminotransferase, serum alkaline phosphatase), total bilirubin, and an albumin should be drawn and monitored daily for 3 to 6 days [22]. N-acetylcysteine (Mucomyst) is the treatment of choice for protecting the liver and preventing methemoglobinemia [22,23]. It works by providing an alternative pathway for the detoxification of acetaminophen or by conjugating the toxic metabolite N-acetyl-p-benzoquinoneimine (NAPQI) [22]. The n-acetylcysteine is diluted to a 5% solution (50 mg/mL) and a loading dose of 140 to 280 mg/kg is administered followed by a maintenance dose of 70 mg/kg every 6 hours for 48 to 72 hours [23]. Other adjunctive treatments include cimetidine (5 to 10 mg/kg PO, SQ every 6 to 9 hours), which may block the hepatic cytochrome that produces the NAPQI [22,23], and ascorbic acid (30 mg/kg PO every 6 to 12 hours) to help reduce any oxidized hemoglobin [22,23].

Venlafaxine

Venlafaxine (Effexor) is a bicyclic antidepressant; it is a serotonin, norepinephrine, and a weak dopamine reuptake inhibitor [25]. Venlafaxine is

overrepresented among medication ingested by ferrets in reports to the
APCC. Previously, it was found that cats, a species that normally does
not voluntarily consume medications, appear to readily ingest venlafaxine
as well [25]. It is possible that there is something in the formulation of the
Effexor that attracts cats and ferrets.

In the APCC database, the lowest recorded dosage in a ferret is 66 mg/kg.
The most common sign seen in ferrets was lethargy or depression. Other
common signs included diarrhea; other CNS changes including hyperactivity, aggression, hyperesthesia, and fasciculations or tremors.

Ingestion of venlafaxine may lead to serotonin syndrome, a condition
caused by elevated levels of serotonin at certain CNS synapses. Initial signs
may be limited to lethargy. However, over time signs such as gastrointestinal
upset, agitation, tremors, hyperthermia, and tachycardia may be seen [26].

Following ingestion of venlafaxine, emesis can be performed in asymptomatic animals. Activated charcoal may be helpful. Since many formulations are extended release, multiple doses of activated charcoal may also
be useful [25]. In addition, since signs may be delayed with extended release
formulations, the ferret should be watched for about 12 hours after the exposure. Once signs begin, cyproheptadine, a serotonin antagonist, may be
helpful in controlling signs at 1.1 mg/kg PO or per rectum [25,26]. In addition, acepromazine or diazepam can be used to control the agitation and
propranolol for the control of the tachycardia [25,26].

Bromethalin

Bromethalin is a rodenticide that affects the CNS [27]. It is not an anticoagulant. It is generally sold as a 0.01% bait. Bromethalin, and its metabolite de-
methylbromethalin, uncouple oxidative phosphorylation especially in the
CNS. This leads to loss of the Na^+-K^+ ATPase pump and the retention of fluid
in the brain and spinal cord, particularly in the myelin sheaths, and elevated
CSF pressure [27]. Signs develop from 24 hours to a few days after ingestion
and start with hind-limb weakness. This then can progress to paresis and paralysis of the hind end, which can ascend and eventually cause paralysis of the
muscles of respiration and death. Seizures may occur terminally [13,27]. Toxic
doses for ferrets are not available. The LD_{50} (median lethal dose) varies by species and falls between 0.25 mg/kg for pigs and up to 5.6 mg/kg for dogs [28].

Because there is no effective treatment of bromethalin toxicosis once the
signs have begun [27], treatment is aimed toward aggressive decontamination. Emesis can be performed within the first 4 hours after exposure; gastric
lavage may also be an option [27,28]. Activated charcoal should be administered. Because it appears that bromethalin undergoes enterohepatic recirculation [27], multiple doses of activated charcoal (3 to 6 doses every
8 hours) should be given.

Once signs have begun, treatment is supportive and symptomatic. Steroids, mannitol, and furosemide have been used but they appear to cause

limited improvement. Further, the animal may rapidly deteriorate after the treatment is stopped [27,28]. Mildly effected animals may recover but this may take days or weeks. Paralysis or seizures generally warrant a grave prognosis [27].

Toxic plants

Many common houseplants may be toxic to ferrets if ingested; ferrets who are allowed outside may encounter garden plants that are also toxic. Even so-called nontoxic plants may cause nonspecific vomiting and diarrhea when eaten. Again, the number of possible toxic plants is beyond the scope of this paper. The APCC's Web site (www.aspca.org/apcc) has links to toxic and nontoxic plants. In addition, a recently published book [29] provides a good review of poisonous plants that ferrets are likely to encounter. Finally, the APCC can be consulted about specific ingestions.

In most cases, treatment of plant toxicoses will be symptomatic and supportive. Emesis can be performed in asymptomatic animals. Activated charcoal may be useful in absorbing plant toxins; multiple doses may be appropriate in large ingestions. Fluid therapy to maintain hydration and an antiemetic may be needed in symptomatic animals.

Paints

Because of their curious nature, ferrets may get into paints while their environment is being painted. It is best to confine the ferret while such jobs are being done. While indoor paints no longer contain significant amounts of lead, some exterior paints may still contain lead as pigments [8]. Houses built before 1973 may still have lead paint indoors. Water-based paints, such as acrylic or latex, are considered to be gastrointestinal and dermal irritants; vomiting may occur with large ingestions [30]. These paints may contain only small amounts of ethylene glycol (generally <5%) so small ingestions are not of concern [30]. Oil- and solvent-based paints and stains can cause gastrointestinal upset with secondary aspiration. Additionally, inhalation of solvents may lead to CNS depression and coma [30].

For dermal exposures to water-based paints, a mild pet shampoo or liquid dishwashing detergent and warm water can be used to aid removal of the paint [30]. Solvents, such as turpentine or mineral spirits, should not be used to remove oil-based paints, as these can cause severe dermal inflammation and chemical burns [31]. Instead, the paint can be removed using vegetable or mineral oil and then the ferret bathed in a liquid dishwashing detergent. Dried paint can either be left to wear off with time or the fur can be clipped to remove it [30].

Following ingestion of paint, dilution can be attempted to reduce the risk of emesis. For large ingestions of water-based paints, emesis may be considered, although the risk of serious systemic signs with most ingestions is low [30]. Because of the risk of aspiration, vomiting should not be induced in oil- or solvent-based paints [30]. Vomiting can usually be managed by giving nothing by mouth for a few hours. In the case of oil-based paints, the ferret should be monitored for signs of aspiration and treated appropriately (oxygen, antibiotics, bronchodilators, and so forth).

Soaps and shampoos

Most soaps such as dish and hand soaps and shampoos are anionic/nonionic surfactants [6]. These are treated in the same way as outlined above in the section on cleaning products.

Summary

The behavior of ferrets may predispose them to toxic exposures and their small size places them at a higher risk of serious intoxications. The treatment of toxicity in ferrets should be approached the same as in any other species. General treatments should be started and, when available, specific therapy for a toxicant should be instituted.

References

[1] Richardson J, Balabuszko R. Managing ferret toxicoses. Exotic DVM 2000;2(4):23–6.

[2] Brown SA. Ferrets: basic anatomy, physiology, and husbandry. In: Quesenberry KE, Carpenter JW, editors. Ferrets, rabbits, and rodents: clinical medicine and surgery. 2nd edition. St. Louis (MO): Saunders; 2004. p. 2–12.

[3] DeClementi C. Prevention and treatment of poisoning. In: Gupta RC, editor. Veterinary toxicology: basic and clinical principles. New York: Elsevier; 2007. p. 1139–58.

[4] Pollock C. Emergency medicine of the ferret. Vet Clin North Am Exot Anim Pract 2007; 10(2):463–500.

[5] Yamashita M, Yamashita M, Tanaka J, et al. Vomiting induction by ipecac syrup in dogs and ferrets. J Toxicol Sci 1997;22(5):409–12.

[6] Oehme FW, Kore AM. Miscellaneous indoor toxicants. In: Peterson ME, Talcott PA, editors. Small animal toxicology. 2nd edition. St Louis (MO): Elsevier Saunders; 2006. p. 223–43.

[7] Richardson J. Bleaches. In: Plumlee KH, editor. Clinical veterinary toxicology. St Louis (MO): Mosby; 2004. p. 142–3.

[8] Dunayer EK. Household hazards. In: Morgan RV, editor. Handbook of small animal practice. 5th edition. St Louis (MO): Saunders Elsevier; 2008. p. 1205–11.

[9] Plumb DC. Sucralfate. In: Plumb's veterinary drug handbook. 5th edition. Ames (IA): Blackwell; 2005. p. 722–3.

[10] Volmer PA. Insecticides and molluscicides: pyrethrins and pyrethroids. In: Plumlee KH, editor. Clinical veterinary toxicology. St Louis (MO): Mosby; 2004. p. 188–90.

[11] Wismer T. Insecticides and molluscicides: novel insecticides. In: Plumlee KH, editor. Clinical veterinary toxicology. St Louis (MO): Mosby; 2004. p. 183–6.

[12] Bough M. Permethrin toxicosis in cats. Veterinary technician 2000;21(9):506–7.

[13] Wickstrom ML, Eason CT. Literature search for mustelid-specific toxicants. Science for Conservation 1999;127E:57–65.

[14] Moorman M, Richardson J, Allen C. Managing toxicosis (3/17/2002 presentation on VSPN). Available at: www.vspn.org/Library/Misc/VSPN_M02055.htm. Accessed October 21, 2007.

[15] Larsen KS, Siggurdsson H, Mencke N. Efficacy of imidacloprid, imidacloprid/permethrin and phoxim for flea control in the Mustelidae (ferrets, mink). Parasitol Res 2005;97:S107–12.

[16] Thrall MA, Hamar DW. Alcohols and glycols. In: Gupta RC, editor. Veterinary toxicology: basic and clinical principles. New York: Elsevier; 2007. p. 605–14.

[17] American Society of Health-System Pharmacists. Ibuprofen. In: McEvot GK, editor. AHFS drug information 2003. Bethesda (MD): American Society of Health-System Pharmacists; 2003. p. 1948–54.

[18] Dunayer E. Ibuprofen toxicosis in dogs, cats, and ferrets. Veterinary medicine 2004;99: 580–6.

[19] Richardson JA, Balabuszko RA. Ibuprofen ingestion in ferrets: 43 cases. January 1995– March 2000. Journal of Veterinary Emergency and Critical Care 2001;11(1):53–9.

[20] Means C. Rodenticides and avicides: anticoagulant rodenticides. In: Plumlee KH, editor. Clinical veterinary toxicology. St Louis (MO): Mosby; 2004. p. 444–6.

[21] Richardson J, Gwaltney-Brant SM. Tips for treating anticoagulant rodenticides toxicity in small mammals. Exotic DVM 2002;4(1):5.

[22] Sellon RK. Acetaminophen. In: Peterson ME, Talcott PA, editors. Small animal toxicology. 2nd edition. St Louis (MO): Saunders Elsevier; 2006. p. 550–8.

[23] Means C. Human medications. In: Morgan RV, editor. Handbook of small animal practice. 5th edition. St Louis (MO): Saunders Elsevier; 2008. p. 1212–9.

[24] O'Connor CE. Evaluation of new toxins for mustelid control. Wellington (New Zealand): Department of Conservation; 2002. Available at: http://www.doc.govt.nz/upload/documents/science-and-technical/DSIS56.pdf. Accessed October 20, 2007.

[25] Merola V, Dunayer E. The 10 most common toxicoses in cats. Veterinary medicine 2006; 101(6):339–42.

[26] Gwaltney-Brant S. Pharmaceuticals: antidepressants. In: Plumlee KH, editor. Clinical veterinary toxicology. St Louis (MO): Mosby; 2004. p. 286–90.

[27] Dunayer E. Bromethalin: the other rodenticide. Veterinary medicine 2003;98(9):732–6.

[28] Gupta RC. Non-anticoagulant rodenticides. In: Gupta RC, editor. Veterinary toxicology: basic and clinical principles. New York: Elsevier; 2007. p. 548–60.

[29] Knight AP. A guide to poisonous house and garden plants. Jackson (WY): Teton New Media; 2006.

[30] Klasco RK, editor. Paint. POISINDEX® System (electronic version). Thomson Micromedex, Greenwood Village, Colorado, USA. Available at: http://www.thomsonhc.com. Accessed October 12, 2007.

[31] Klasco RK, editor. Hydrocarbons. POISINDEX® System (electronic version). Thomson Micromedex, Greenwood Village, Colorado, USA. Available at: http://www.thomsonhc.com. Accessed October 12, 2007.

ELSEVIER
SAUNDERS

VETERINARY
CLINICS
Exotic Animal Practice

Vet Clin Exot Anim 11 (2008) 315–326

Clinical Toxicoses of Domestic Rabbits

Matthew S. Johnston, VMD, DABVP–Avian*

*James L. Voss Veterinary Teaching Hospital, Colorado State University,
300 West Drake Road, Fort Collins, CO 80523, USA*

Toxicoses are an uncommon presentation to rabbit practitioners; however, veterinarians who accept rabbits as patients should be familiar with the basic concepts of toxicosis management and the specific syndromes associated with clinical toxicoses. The objective of this article is to present clinically relevant information for veterinarians presented with rabbits exhibiting characteristic signs of toxicosis. In addition, specific mention is made to the most common clinical toxicoses, including lead, chemicals, rodenticides, aflatoxins, and poisonous plants.

Decontamination

In the case of acute, known toxin exposure, similar guidelines to detoxification of other small animals can be used. In the event of topical exposure of a known or potential toxin, rabbits should be bathed using a mild shampoo solution, and eyes should be copiously lavaged with sterile saline. Normal rabbits rapidly groom any foreign substance off their hair coat, so attention should be paid to the possibility of ingestion in addition to topical exposure. When bathing rabbits, one must use caution to prevent injury to the patient. Ideally, rabbits are bathed in a vessel that approximates their body size, such as a laundry sink, using a spray nozzle. The rabbit should be restrained by an assistant during the bath to prevent injury. Water temperature should be warm (102°F–105°F) and the shampoo or soap solution chosen should be a mild puppy/kitten or baby shampoo. When shampooing, one should take care to not only wash the fur but also massage the shampoo down to the level of the skin to remove any toxin that may have penetrated deeply through the pelage. After rinsing, the rabbit should be towel-dried immediately and placed into a warm cage to complete drying. Monitoring

* James L. Voss Veterinary Teaching Hospital, 300 West Drake Road, Fort Collins, CO 80523.
   E-mail address: msjohn@colostate.edu

of body temperature is critical because hyperthermia due to hot air dryers and hypothermia due to evaporative cooling occurs easily and quickly. Early signs of hyperthermia (axillary temperature > 102.5°F) include vaso-dilation of the auricular vessels, nasal flare, and rapid respiratory rate. Early signs of hypothermia (axillary temperature < 100°F) include shivering, pale mucus membranes, and a compact body posture. External cooling with fans or heating with forced warm air blowers, circulating hot water blankets, or heating pads is recommended to maintain the body temperature between 100°F and 102.5°F until the rabbit is dry and able to thermoregulate efficiently on its own.

When the route of toxin ingestion is oral, decontamination is more challenging in rabbits than in dogs or cats. Rabbits cannot vomit, making gastric decontamination by way of emetics impossible. Gastric lavage can be used in certain situations to reduce the amount of toxins that are pre-sented to the jejunum for absorption. Gastric lavage is contraindicated in rabbits that are too unstable to handle anesthesia because anesthesia and endotracheal intubation are required to safely perform the technique. The procedure should be performed with extreme caution in rabbits that have ingested petroleum distillates because these chemicals can induce a severe and usually fatal tracheitis, bronchitis, and pneumonitis if allowed to enter the respiratory tree. Finally, gastric lavage is contraindicated when any caustic substance that may cause worsening of esophageal ulceration during lavage has been ingested [1].

Rabbits must be anesthetized and endotracheally intubated for this proce-dure. Endotracheal intubation is necessary to protect the airway; however, aspiration of lavage contents is still possible, so some investigators have recommended this technique only when potentially lethal substances have been ingested [1]. If the potential toxin ingestion occurred within 24 hours of presentation, then gastric lavage will likely be of some benefit because gastric emptying can be slow in rabbits, especially those that are ill. A com-bination of ketamine (2–5 mg/kg) and midazolam (0.25–0.5 mg/kg) given in-travenously usually induces adequate anesthesia for endotracheal intubation. Other induction agents and the techniques for endotracheal intubation have been described elsewhere [2]. An orogastric tube of large diameter (8–16 Fr in most rabbits) is chosen, and the rabbit is placed in left lateral recumbency. After the rabbit is endotracheally intubated, a flexible tube is measured to the level of the ninth intercostal space, lubricated with water-soluble lubri-cant, and passed orally until it reaches the stomach. Resistance may be met at the level of the lower esophageal sphincter but is usually easily over-come by rotating the tube or instilling a small amount of air through it while applying gentle pressure. A warmed lavage solution of water or 0.9% saline is instilled by way of the tube at a volume of approximately 10 mL/kg. The stomach contents are agitated by way of external massage, and the lavage solution is then reaspirated. In most cases, a fair amount of lavage fluid will leak around the tube into the esophagus, so the rabbit's head should be placed in a dependent position to prevent pooling of fluid in the back of the oropharynx and to decrease the risk of aspiration. This procedure generally needs to be repeated 10 to 15 times to gain maximal decontamination. Gastric rupture, gastric ulceration, esophagitis, esophageal ulceration, and aspiration are the main risks associated with this procedure.

Activated charcoal can then be infused by way of the orogastric tube to adsorb remaining toxicants. Activated charcoal acts by directly adsorbing the toxicant from the gastrointestinal (GI) tract, interrupting enterohepatic circulation, and enhancing the rate of diffusion of chemicals from the body into the GI tract [3]. Activated charcoal should be used following gastric lavage in cases of known or suspected ingestion of organic poisons, bacterial toxins, pesticides, rodenticides, mercuric chloride, strychnine and anesthetic alkaloids (morphine, atropine), barbiturates, and ethylene glycol. Activated charcoal is not indicated in the known or suspected ingestion of cyanide, heavy metals, or caustic materials [1]. A dose of 1 to 3 g/kg in a concentration of 1 g per 5 to 10 mL of water has been reported [1,3]. In most instances, redosing every 4 to 8 hours for 24 hours is beneficial. For subsequent doses, if the rabbit is stable and swallowing, the activated charcoal can be administered by way of a syringe. Sodium sulfate and sorbitol cathartics are commonly combined with activated charcoal in commercial preparations, although no reports exist of their use in rabbits. Because of this, these preparations should be used with caution, if used at all, because they may predispose to diarrhea and increased fluid loss.

A final step in preventing further absorption of toxins in rabbits is the application of an Elizabethan collar to prevent ingestion of cecotrophs that may contain toxic residues [1]. The Elizabethan collar should be left on for 72 hours following initial absorption to ensure that cecotrophs are free of toxicants.

Elimination of most toxins is generally achieved by way of the kidneys, although other routes may also be important. To enhance elimination, diuresis by way of intravenous administration of balanced crystalloids at a rate of 4 to 8 mL/kg/h is indicated in most cases. When intravenous access is not possible, the subcutaneous route of fluid administration can result in adequate diuresis. In toxins with fecal or biliary elimination, forced feedings may be beneficial in aiding in decontamination. Generally, 10 to 20 mL/kg of an appropriate herbivore feeding formula administered 3 to 6 times daily produces adequate fecal output.

Lead toxicosis

Lead toxicosis is a common toxicosis of pet rabbits. Lead paint contamination of houses built prior to 1974 is the most common cause of intoxication, although golf balls, improperly glazed ceramics, linoleum glue, metallic objects containing lead, and lead soldering are other possibilities. Historically, rabbits that have lead toxicosis commonly chew at baseboards or plasterboards, so the age of the house in question should be determined. Lead paint stopped being used in the United States in 1974, whereas lead pipes were outlawed in 1984. In many older homes, these lead pipes are still readily accessible in unfinished basements.

The most common clinical presentation of lead toxicosis in rabbits is hyporexia progressing to anorexia; however, other signs including behavioral changes; neurologic abnormalities such as seizures, torticollis, and blindness; and chronic loss of body condition have been seen [4–6]. Physical examination may also reveal cardiac arrhythmias as a result of myocarditis or intimal hypertrophy [7,8] and hypertension due to interference with the renin-angiotensin system [9,10]. Although plasma biochemical testing is usually unremarkable in rabbits that have lead toxicosis, hematologic changes such as anemia with a reticulocytosis and nucleated erythrocytes, hypochromasia, poikilocytosis, anisocytosis, and basophilic stippling of the erythrocytes occur with some frequency but are not specific or sensitive for lead toxicosis [5,8,11]. Chronic lead toxicosis is also known to contribute to immunosuppression in rabbits [12], possibly through the induction of a neutropenia [5,11]. In one clinical case report, an intoxicated rabbit presented with a neutropenia (presumed to be a heteropenia) and subsequently died of pneumonia following treatment for lead toxicosis [4]. In this case, the heterophil count was never repeated, so it is unknown whether it persisted and possibly predisposed this rabbit to develop pneumonia.

The definitive diagnosis of lead toxicosis is based on blood lead concentrations. Because lead is not a normal constituent of the body, theoretically, no lead should be detectable in the blood; however, normal blood lead concentrations of less than 22 µg/dL and 2 to 27 µg/dL have been reported in the literature [5,13]. Toxicosis has been defined as greater than 30 µg/dL [5], and two rabbits reported in the literature that had clinical lead toxicosis had values of 70 µg/dL and 40 µg/dL [4]. Treatment is recommended for any rabbit that has a concentration of blood lead greater than 10 µg/dL (the lower limit of detection for most assays) because clinical signs have been seen at concentrations less than the classically defined toxicosis concentration. Furthermore, blood lead concentrations do not correlate with the severity of clinical signs because they fluctuate based on chronicity of exposure and the form of lead ingested [5,14,15].

When a definitive diagnosis has been made based on blood lead concentrations, abdominal radiographs are indicated to assess for the presence of metallic opacities within the GI tract, because these may represent the source of lead. Although lubricant laxatives were used in the published case report of rabbits that had lead toxicosis [4], they are probably not necessary as long as management of the ileus generally associated with lead toxicosis is implemented. Subcutaneous balanced crystalloids and force feeding of 10 to 20 mL/kg of an appropriate herbivore diet usually moves any metallic objects through the GI tract in 2 to 3 days. Metal analysis of the objects recovered in the feces may be warranted if the owner is unsure of the source. Radiographs should be repeated periodically until all metallic opacities are shown to have passed.

The recommended treatment for rabbits that have lead toxicosis, as in other mammals, is chelation with calcium-EDTA. Calcium-EDTA works by chelating lead from the bones and presenting it to the kidneys for excretion. Lead is subsequently removed from soft tissues as its concentration equilibrates with that of the bones [16]. The recommended dose in dogs, which was used successfully in the published case report of the two rabbits that had lead toxicosis, is 27.5 mg/kg administered subcutaneously every 6 hours for 2 to 5 days [4,14]. A dose of 30 mg/kg administered subcutaneously every 12 hours for 5 to 7 days has also been used successfully by the author in multiple cases, and the twice-daily dosing is more practical for pet owners. Blood lead concentrations should be rechecked 5 to 7 days after stopping chelation, which allows time for soft tissue lead concentrations to equilibrate with bone. Most rabbits require more than one course of chelation to bring the blood lead concentration to below 10 μg/dL. It is recommended that any lead present in the GI tract be removed prior to beginning chelation therapy because chelators enhance GI absorption of lead and may worsen clinical signs initially [17]. The use of oral chelators has not been reported in rabbits. It is important to also provide nutritional support by way of force feedings to rabbits that have lead toxicosis because most are hyporexic or anorexic on presentation. Other supportive care is implemented as indicated by the presenting clinical signs (ie, administration of diazepam or midazolam to control seizures, lubrication of eyes, and treatment of corneal ulcers in severe cases of torticollis).

In the event of a fatal lead toxicosis, heavy metal analysis of stomach or cecal contents may help to establish a definitive diagnosis. Histopathologic lesions consistent with lead toxicosis include myocardial degeneration, multifocal hepatic necrosis, renal tubular degeneration, and renal tubules that contain hemoglobin casts [17]. Heart blood can also be used for lead concentration analysis.

The final consideration in the management of lead toxicosis is removal of the source of lead or prevention of access to the source of lead. In the case of an identifiable object, this object should be removed from the reach of the rabbit. In the case of lead paint ingestion, barricades to the walls, baseboards, or plasterboards should be put permanently in place anywhere the rabbit is allowed to roam. Metal adjustable outdoor dog fencing works well as a rabbit barrier and is flexible enough to suit the shape of most rooms. Owners of rabbits should also be counseled to monitor rabbits for licking or chewing at walls and to discourage this behavior as much as possible.

Chemicals

For decades, rabbits have been used as laboratory models for toxicity studies of various chemicals. A review of this entire body of literature is beyond the scope of this manuscript; however, the practitioner should be aware in the case of suspected or known exposure of a rabbit to a medical, cosmetic, or hygienic chemical that there is likely to be some literature available for consultation. A good review of effects of commonly used external agents (shampoos, hair dyes, cosmetics, and so forth) is available, although it is somewhat dated and does not include newer products [18]. Some pharmaceutics commonly used by veterinarians are known to cause toxic effects in rabbits, and a discussion of these chemicals is included here.

Fipronil (Frontline) is registered for use as an ectoparasiticide on dogs and cats. Although its successful use has been reported in rabbits [19,20], multiple reports exist of young or small rabbits that were intentionally dosed with fipronil and, within 24 hours, exhibited signs of anorexia and lethargy with or without seizures, or died [20]. In the event of known accidental or intentional application of fipronil to a rabbit, the rabbit should be treated as outlined earlier for topical cutaneous exposure. In addition, the use of activated charcoal may be indicated in these cases because rabbits rapidly groom off any product applied topically, so ingestion of fipronil is likely. When a rabbit already shows clinical signs, prognosis for recovery is guarded. Bathing and activated charcoal should still be attempted to limit any additional absorption of the drug. Supportive care consisting of diuresis, force feeding, and control of seizures with midazolam or diazepam is given in the hope that the rabbit will recover. If there is no improvement in the first 72 hours, then it is unlikely that exposed rabbit will recover.

There are conflicting reports in the literature of the renal toxicity of D-limonene to rabbits, with one source listing it as toxic [1] and others suggest that it is not [21,22]. The limonenes are monocyclic monoterpenes found in orange peel and other plants that are commonly used to fragrance household products [22]. They have been recommended for use in laboratory rabbits for large-volume blood collection because of their vasodilatory effects [21]. D-Limonene is known to be toxic to male rats, and this toxicity is thought to be related to a high expression of α2u-globulin in the liver of male rats. Male rats express approximately 100 times more α2u-globulin in their livers than female rats, and many chemicals, including the limonenes, induce renal toxicity by reversibly binding to α2u-globulin after it has been secreted from the liver. This binding prevents hydrolysis of proteins, thereby causing accumulation of protein droplets in the renal tubules, resulting in failure [23]. Differences in the metabolism of limonenes between rabbits and other species, however, suggest that D-limonene is nontoxic in rabbits [22,24]. It is likely that the initial report of its toxicity in rabbits was a result of extrapolation from other well-studied species.

When applied in high concentrations, permethrin or pyrethrin sprays or spot-on products are reportedly toxic to rabbits [1] and may cause anorexia, lethargy, twitching, and seizures. A commercial pyrethroid, cypermethrin, has been shown to induce biochemical and hematologic changes such as hyperlipidemia, hypercholesterolemia, hyperglycemia, azotemia, hyperbilirubinemia, hypoproteinemia, low hemoglobin concentration, and leukocytosis [25]. Although a clinical report of the successful use of these chemicals exists in the literature, this report does not detail the dose given [26]. There are over 10,000 commercial formulations containing almost 450 different pesticidal pyrethroids [25], so it is impossible to detail the potential toxicities and treatment of suspected or confirmed toxicoses of all of them. In addition to the decontamination steps discussed earlier, there is mounting evidence in various species that antioxidants such as vitamins C and E, β-carotene [27,28], zinc, selenium [29], and isoflavones [30] may help reduce some of the toxic effects of pyrethroids. With the reported safety and efficacy of selamectin (Revolution) in rabbits, this product has replaced many pyrethrins and permethrins in addition to fipronil for the treatment by veterinarians of ectoparasites in rabbits [31,32]. Pyrethrins and permethrins are still available over-the-counter for pet owners as spot-on or spray-on applications and are widely used in agriculture and home-use pesiticide applications, so education of rabbit owners about the possible risks associated with the use of these products should be provided.

Other pesticides such as organophosphates have fallen out of favor since the introduction of the relatively safer pyrethroids, but organophosphate toxicosis is still possible in domestic rabbits allowed to graze outdoors. Rabbits that have organophosphate toxicosis show clinical signs as a result of cholinesterase inhibition, such as drooling, lacrimation, urination, and muscle weakness. The relevance to this clinical discussion is that many rabbits have intrinsic atropinesterases [2]. Atropine is traditionally used as an antidote to organophosphate toxicants, and the presence of these atropinesterases may preclude its effective use in rabbits. In place of or in addition to atropine, the oxime pralidoxime chloride (2-PAM) is effective at reversing the signs associated with organophosphate toxicosis [33,34].

Macrolide and β-lactam antibiotics are well documented to cause a potentially fatal typhlitis in rabbits, although it is likely the effects are more a result of disruption of the normal cecal flora and not a direct toxic effect of the antibiotics [35,36]. Aminoglycosides such as gentamicin, amikacin, and streptomycin, on the other hand, have a direct nephrotoxic effect [35,37]. All aminoglycosides have the potential to induce acute tubular necrosis and should therefore be used only when culture and sensitivity results indicate. In rabbits being given gentamicin, supplementation with vitamin B_6 (pyridoxine) at 10 mg per rabbit was shown to be an effective preventative measure for the development of gentamicin-induced acute tubular necrosis [38].

The anesthetic combination of tiletamine and zolazepam (Telazol) has been shown to cause acute renal failure characterized by azotemia, proteinuria, and the presence of tubular casts within 24 hours of intramuscular injection (20, 32, and 64 mg/kg). In these reports, severe renal tubular necrosis was evident on histopathologic examination [39,40]. Tiletamine/zolazepam combinations are contraindicated in rabbits. The toxic principle of this combination in rabbits has not been worked out.

Rodenticides

Anticoagulant rodenticides such as warfarin, difenacoum, and brodifacoum are still widely available for home and industrial use. Although homes containing rabbits should not use these rodenticides, accidental toxicoses still occur with some regularity. Clinical signs of anticoagulant rodenticides in rabbits are similar to those seen in other small animals and characterized by bleeding into body cavities due to inhibition of vitamin K_1 epoxide reductase [1,41]. The newer generation of anticoagulant rodenticides (difenacoum and brodifacoum) may have effects that last as long as 20 days in the rabbit, necessitating long treatment regimens [42]. Clinical signs following oral ingestion generally occur within 24 to 72 hours. In the case of known or suspected ingestion prior to the onset of clinical signs, gastric lavage followed by activated charcoal administration as described earlier is indicated. When clinical signs are already apparent or when prolongation in clotting times or the presence of PIVKA proteins (proteins induced by vitamin K absence of antagonists) [43] is apparent on laboratory analysis of coagulation, gastric lavage and activated charcoal are likely of little clinical utility.

Initial stabilization of the bleeding rabbit consists of fresh whole blood transfusions to provide clotting factors and to stabilize the total protein and packed cell volume. Specific blood group antigens have not been described for rabbits, so an in-house major cross-match should be performed [1]. After blood is obtained from a donor rabbit, one drop of plasma from the recipient is mixed with one drop of blood from the donor on a glass slide. If any evidence of agglutination occurs during mixing, then the donor blood should not be administered because a transfusion reaction would likely occur. While this transfusion is being prepared, injectable vitamin K_1 should be administered. Published doses range from 2 to 12 mg/kg given intramuscularly (subcutaneous and intravenous doses have been associated with anaphylaxis) [1,44]. Following stabilization, oral vitamin K_1 therapy should be continued for 1 to 4 weeks (longer for newer-generation rodenticides) [1]. The most practical way to administer vitamin K_1 orally is to use the injectable form, although its effects may take up to 18 hours to begin working [44]. Oral bioavailability is enhanced by the concurrent administration of a small amount of fat, so owners are often instructed to give the vitamin with a teaspoonful of corn or vegetable oil.

Clinical toxicosis and research studies in rabbits of the newer rodenticides, including bromethalin and cholecalciferol, are scarce in the literature. The median lethal dose of bromethalin is known to be 13 mg/kg in the rabbit, which is approximately 3 times that of the dog and 10 times that of the cat [45]. The most common commercial products containing bromethalin have a concentration of 0.01% (0.1 mg/g) bromethalin [45], which means that a large amount ($\sim$390 g) would need to be consumed by the average 3-kg rabbit to reach lethal doses. This large amount likely explains the lack of reported cases; furthermore, it appears that bromethalin might be a safer alternative to anticoagulant rodenticides for homes in which rabbits reside. Briefly, bromethalin acts by causing uncoupling of oxidative phosphorylation in the central nervous system and liver mitochondria, resulting in decreased ATP and alterations in the sodium/potassium ATPase. By way of inability to maintain osmotic gradients, intracranial pressure due to cerebral edema increases, causing clinical signs of central nervous system disease and, ultimately, death [45].

Cholecalciferol is vitamin D_3, which is bioactivated to calcitriol. Calcitriol causes a marked increase in plasma calcium levels, leading to metastatic calcification and acute renal failure. Cholecalciferol rodenticides are likely fatal in rabbits, and treatment would be similar to that in other animals, although there is an absence of research studies or clinical reports in the literature.

Aflatoxins

Aflatoxicosis was first experimentally induced in rabbits in 1980 [46], although the first clinical report appeared in 1973 [47]. Aflatoxins are secondary metabolites of fungus, namely *Aspergillus* spp. Although there are several known toxins, aflatoxin B_1 is the most clinically important. Aflatoxicosis is best prevented by the purchase of feedstuffs from reputable retailers and the proper (dry, cool, short-term) storage of hay and chow. The disease appears rarely and can be very difficult to definitively diagnose due to the chronicity of signs. Young animals are more readily affected than mature animals [48].

Clinical signs of aflatoxicosis are vague and include hyporexia, lethargy and dull mental status, decreased water consumption, slow weight gain in growing animals, and slow mortalities in rabbitries. Definitive diagnosis is by a combination of characteristic histopathologic lesions including focal hepatic necrosis with dilation and engorgement of sinusoids; biliary hyperplasia, periportal fibrosis, and mononuclear inflammation; renal tubular degeneration and mononuclear inflammation; myocardial degeneration; and demonstration of elevated aflatoxin levels in feed [49]. The median lethal dose for aflatoxins of rabbits is among the lowest of all species studied [46], and levels as low as 2 ppm aflatoxin in feed are likely to cause clinical problems [48].

Poisonous plants

As grazing herbivores, rabbits commonly ingest household and garden plants. Although most of these plants do not cause any problems, some may be toxic to rabbits. In most cases, rabbit-specific toxicity is unknown, so when a plant is known to be toxic to another species, it should be assumed to be toxic to rabbits unless proven otherwise. An exhaustive report of every poisonous plant that a rabbit may ingest is beyond the scope of this manuscript; however, an excellent recently published resource for veterinarians and rabbit owners is available that provides a nearly comprehensive review of this topic, including common and scientific names, photographs of leaves and fruit, toxic principles and mechanisms of action, risk assessment, clinical signs of toxicosis, and treatment [50].

Rabbit owners should be instructed to bring samples of the leaves and fruits of plants suspected of having been ingested if the name or genus/species of the plant is not known. The veterinarian can then use Internet resources or the previously mentioned reference to help identify the plant and determine toxicity. Treatment is generally aimed at decontamination (as highlighted earlier) and specific treatment depending on the toxic principle and mechanism of action (ie, gastric and esophageal protectants in the case of ingestion of oxalate-containing plants). Rabbit owners should always be questioned historically about the possibility of plant ingestion in rabbits that have undiagnosed syndromes to see whether a poisonous plant may have been responsible. Plant ingestion is best prevented by supervised grazing outdoors or by removal of plants from the rabbit's environment.

References

[1] Oglesbee BL. Poisoning (intoxication). In: Oglesbee BL, editor. The 5-minute veterinary consult: ferret and rabbit. Ames (IA): Blackwell; 2006. p. 324–5.

[2] Heard DJ. Anesthesia, analgesia, and sedation of small mammals. In: Quesenberry KE, Carpenter JW, editors. Ferrets, rabbits, and rodents: clinical medicine and surgery. 2nd edition. St. Louis (MO): Saunders; 2004. p. 356–69.

[3] Ofoefule SI, Onuoha LC, Okonta MJ, et al. Effect of activated charcoal on isoniazid absorption in rabbits. Boll Chim Farm 2001;140(3):183–6.

[4] Swartout MS, Gerken DF. Lead-induced toxicosis in two domestic rabbits. J Am Vet Med Assoc 1987;191(6):717–9.

[5] Roscoe DE, Nielsen SW, Eaton HD, et al. Chronic plumbism in rabbits: a comparison of three diagnostic tests. Am J Vet Res 1975;36:1225–9.

[6] Deeb BJ, Carpenter JW. Neurological and musculoskeletal diseases. In: Quesenberry KE, Carpenter JW, editors. Ferrets, rabbits, and rodents: clinical medicine and surgery. 2nd edition. St. Louis (MO): Saunders; 2004. p. 203–10.

[7] Stofen D. Environmental lead and the heart. J Mol Cell Cardiol 1974;6:285–90.

[8] Bartlett RS, Rousseau JE, Frier HI, et al. Effect of vitamin E on delta-aminolevulinic acid dehydratase activity in weanling rabbits with chronic plumbism. J Nutr 1974;104: 1637–45.

[9] Beevers DG, Erskine E, Robertson M, et al. Blood-lead and hypertension. Lancet 1976;308: 1–3.

[10] Mouw DR, Vander AJ, Cox J, et al. Acute effects of lead on renal electrolyte excretion and plasma renin activity. Toxicol Appl Pharmacol 1978;46:435–47.

[11] Haas GM, Brown DVL, Eisenstein R, et al. Relations between lead poisoning in rabbit and man. Am J Pathol 1964;45:691–715.

[12] Koller LD. Immunosuppression produced by lead, cadmium and mercury. Am J Vet Res 1973;34:1457–8.

[13] Gerken DF, Swartout MS. Blood lead concentrations in rabbits. Am J Vet Res 1986;47: 2674–5.

[14] Kowalcyk DF. Clinical management of lead poisoning. J Am Vet Med Assoc 1984;184: 858–60.

[15] Johnson JH, Dollahite JW. Comparison of the oral lethality of lead acetate and lead carbonate in rabbits. Am J Vet Res 1978;39:1241.

[16] Doniec J, Trojanowska B, Trzcinka-Ochocka M, et al. Effects of Na2Ca EDTA on lead deposits in rabbit osseous tissue. Toxicol Lett 1983;19:1–5.

[17] Percy DH, Barthold SW. Rabbits. In: Percy DH, Barthold SW, editors. Pathology of laboratory rodents and rabbits. Ames (IA): Iowa State Press; 2001. p. 248–306.

[18] Stenbäck F. Local and systemic effects of commonly used cutaneous agents: lifetime studies of 16 compounds in mice and rabbits. Acta Pharmacol Toxicol (Copenh) 1977;41: 417–31.

[19] Cutler SL. Ectopic Psoroptes cuniculi infestation in a pet rabbit. J Small Anim Pract 1998;39: 86–7.

[20] Cooper PE, Penaliggon J. Use of Frontline spray on rabbits. Vet Rec 1997;140:535–6.

[21] Lacy MJ, Kent CR, Voss EW. D-Limonene: an effective vasodilator for use in collecting rabbit blood. Lab Anim Sci 1987;37(4):485–7.

[22] Shimada T, Shindo M, Miyazawa M. Species differences in the metabolism of (+)- and (−)-limonenes and their metabolites, carveols and carvones, by cytochrome P450 enzymes in liver microsomes of mice, rats, guinea pigs, rabbits, dogs, monkeys, and humans. Drug Metab Pharmacokinet 2002;17(6):507–15.

[23] Lehman-Mckeeman LD, Rodriquez PA, Takigiku R, et al. D-Limonene-induced male rat-specific nephrotoxicity: evaluation of the association between D-limonene and α2u-globulin. Toxicol Appl Pharmacol 1989;99:250–9.

[24] Kanerva RL, Alden CL. Review of kidney sections from a subchronic D-limonene oral dosing study conducted by the National Cancer Institute. Food Chem Toxicol 1987;25: 355–8.

[25] Yousef MI, El-Demerdash FM, Kamel KI, et al. Changes in some hematological and biochemical indices of rabbits induced by isoflavones and cypermethrin. Toxicol 2003;189: 223–34.

[26] Pinter L. Leporacarus gibbus and Spilopsyllus cuniculi infestation in a pet rabbit. J Small Anim Pract 1999;40:220–1.

[27] Bagchi D, Bagchi M, Stohs SJ, et al. Free radicals and grape seed proanthocyanidin extract: importance in human health and disease prevention. Toxicol 2000;148:187–97.

[28] Yousef MI, El-Demerdash FM, El-Agamy EI. Effect of ascorbic acid on some biochemical parameters of rabbits affected by aflatoxin B1. Environ Nut Intl 1999;3(3):141–53.

[29] Pregiosi P, Galan P, Hebeth B, et al. Effect of supplementation with a combination of antioxidant vitamins and trace elements, at nutritional doses, on biochemical indicators and markers of the antioxidant system in adult subjects. J Am Coll Nutr 1998;17(3):244–9.

[30] El-Demerdash FM, Yousef MI, Al-Salhen KS. Protective effects of isoflavone on some biochemical parameters affected by cypermethrin in male rabbits. J Environ Sci Health B 2003; B38(3):365–78.

[31] McTier TL, Hair JA, Walstrom DJ, et al. Efficacy and safety of topical administration of selamectin for treatment of ear mite infestation in rabbits. J Am Vet Med Assoc 2003; 223(3):322–4.

[32] Kurtdede A, Karaer Z, Acar A, et al. Use of selamectin for the treatment of psoroptic and sarcoptic mite infestation in rabbits. Vet Dermatol 2007;18(1):18–22.

[33] Bevandic Z, Deljac A, Makisimovic M, et al. Methylthio analogues of PAM-2, TMB-4, and obidoxime as antidotes in organophosphate poisonings. Acta Pharm Jugosl 1985;35: 213–8.

[34] Koplovitz I, Stewart JR. A comparison of the efficacy of HI6 and 2-PAM against soman, tabun, sarin, and VX in the rabbit. Toxicol Lett 1994;70:269–79.

[35] Harkness JE, Wagner JE. Clinical procedures. In: Harkness JE, Wagner JE, editors. The biology and medicine of rabbits and rodents. Media. Pennsylvania: Williams and Wilkins; 1995. p. 75–142.

[36] Jenkins JR. Gastrointestinal diseases. In: Quesenberry KE, Carpenter JW, editors. Ferrets, rabbits, and rodents: clinical medicine and surgery. 2nd edition. St. Louis (MO): Saunders; 2004. p. 161–71.

[37] Kojima T, Kabayashi T, Iwase S, et al. Gentamicin nephrotoxicity in young rabbits. Exp Pathol 1984;26:71–5.

[38] Enriquez JI, Schydlower M, O'Hair K, et al. Effect of vitamin B_6 supplementation on gentamicin nephrotoxicity in rabbits. Vet Hum Toxicol 1992;34(1):32–5.

[39] Evans KD, Dillehay DL, Huerkamp MJ, et al. Diagnostic exercise: azotemia in a rabbit (*Oryctolagus cuniculus*). Lab Anim Sci 1996;46(4):442–3.

[40] Brammer DW, Doerning BJ, Chrisp CE, et al. Anesthetic and nephrotoxic effects of Telazol in New Zealand white rabbits. Lab Anim Sci 1991;41(5):432–5.

[41] Winn MJ, Cholerton S, Park BK. An investigation of the pharmacological response to vitamin K_1 in the rabbit. Br J Pharmacol 1988;94:1077–84.

[42] Breckenridge AM, Cholerton JAD, Hart BK, et al. A study of the relationship between the pharmacokinetics and the pharmacodynamics of the 4-hydroxycoumarin anticoagulants warfarin, difenacoum and brodifacoum in the rabbit. Br J Pharmacol 1985;84:81–91.

[43] Zivelin A, Vijaya Mohan Rao L, Rapaport SI. Plasma PIVKA proteins in rabbits given warfarin. Thromb Res 1996;82(5):429–38.

[44] Nagata M, Yotsuyanagi T, Nonomura M, et al. Coagulation recovery after warfarin-induced hypoprothrombinaemia by oral administration of liposomally-associated vitamin K_1 to rabbits. J Pharm Pharmacol 1984;36:527–33.

[45] van Lier RB, Cherry LD. The toxicity and mechanism of action of bromethalin: a new single-feeding rodenticide. Fundam Appl Toxicol 1988;11(4):664–72.

[46] Clark JD, Jain AV, Hatch RC, et al. Experimentally induced chronic aflatoxicosis in rabbits. Am J Vet Res 1980;41(11):1841–5.

[47] Mehotra ML, Khanna RS. Aflatoxicosis in Angora rabbits. Indian Vet J 1973;50:620–2.

[48] Makkar HPS, Singh B. Aflatoxicosis in rabbits. J Appl Rabbit Res 1991;14:218–21.

[49] Krishna L, Dawra RK, Vaid J, et al. An outbreak of aflatoxicosis in Angora rabbits. Vet Hum Toxicol 1991;33(2):159–61.

[50] Knight AP. A guide to poisonous house and garden plants. Jackson (WY): Teton NewMedia; 2006.

ELSEVIER
SAUNDERS

VETERINARY
CLINICS
Exotic Animal Practice

Vet Clin Exot Anim 11 (2008) 327–357

Poisonings in Reptiles

Kevin T. Fitzgerald, PhD, DVM, DABVP*,
Kristin L. Newquist, BS, AAS, CVT

Alameda East Veterinary Hospital, Denver, CO 80231, USA

"Sometimes even a snake needs a doctor."
—Groucho Marx

Humans are potentially at risk for exposure to an ever-growing array of toxic substances. Environmental sources, industrial molecules, pesticides and herbicides, over-the-counter and prescription pharmaceuticals, even human diets generate a constantly expanding number of possible toxins. Other life forms are by no means immune to these hazards and often are equally susceptible to the increasing body of potential poisons. In particular, domestic animals, companion species, and animals kept in zoologic collections have become increasingly at risk.

In recent years, nontraditional, "exotic" species have become increasingly popular household pets. Veterinarians therefore must contend with an ever-broadening number of poisons and also must learn the biology, natural history, medical treatment, and physiologic idiosyncrasies of an ever-enlarging number of species. This broadening scope is particularly apparent in the widening number of reptile species presented to veterinary hospitals and animal emergency rooms. Veterinarians are in a cruel bind: they must become familiar with more and more species, and they also must be able to identify and treat a burgeoning number of toxic molecules.

Practitioners cannot be expected to be familiar with every hazardous substance, but clinicians must understand that toxicology is an essential part of emergency medicine, and they must come to recognize the most commonly presented toxidromes. Veterinarians treating exotic patients must strive to keep current as new information both about these species and about new poisonings becomes available. The veterinary practitioner is duty bound to provide state-of-the-art medical care to all patients, including nontraditional exotics, and the standard of care is changing constantly as the level of knowledge concerning these animals grows. Veterinarians must keep learning.

---
* Corresponding author.
E-mail address: kfitzgerald@aevh.com (K.T. Fitzgerald).

1094-9194/08/$ - see front matter © 2008 Elsevier Inc. All rights reserved.
doi:10.1016/j.cvex.2008.01.004   *vetexotic.theclinics.com*

Intoxication of reptiles by various poisons was once an almost exclusively anecdotal domain. For too long these cases merely "fell through the slats." In the last 10 years, however, with the development of animal poison hot lines, the improvement of toxicology curricula in veterinary schools, the efforts of the American Board of Veterinary Toxicology, and a large number of outlets publishing both case histories and the results of in-depth pharmacologic studies, the knowledge of poisonings in reptiles has blossomed significantly. This article focuses on the most common poisonings, their mechanism of action, and their care and treatment in captive and wild reptiles.

Emergency medicine for poisoned reptiles

Veterinarians must become accustomed to approaching any intoxicated animal in a systematic fashion and must work up these cases in exotic species just as they would in any critically ill animal. To maximize the possibility of a favorable outcome, poisoning cases must be managed swiftly and rigorously from the initial telephone call or presentation. Receptionists, technicians, and all hospital support staff must be trained and educated in dealing with toxicologic emergencies. Support staffs are only as capable and competent as they are allowed to be. In-house training sessions for staff regarding poisons are tremendously effective and can provide spectacular benefits. Helping staff recognize what can be deadly and what is harmless can make the difference between life and death. Thus for the successful management of toxicologic cases the telephone is the first line of defense. Boxes 1 and 2 summarize the most pertinent points for veterinarians and staff concerning the initial telephone contact and taking a toxicologic history. Box 3 includes a sample toxicology history form.

Many reptile owners know very little about the exotic animal they keep in their home. As a result, emergency situations in their reptile are not always obvious to them. Likewise, many veterinarians are not familiar enough with anatomy, physiology, and vital signs of these captive reptile species. Furthermore, like many other wild animals, captive reptiles do much to mask the outward signs of disease. Nevertheless, the practicing exotic clinician must understand that the basic tenets of emergency medicine remain the same, regardless of the species involved. Although when exotic species become ill they present special diagnostic challenges to practitioners, and although reptiles can become accidentally poisoned in a variety of ways, the clinician can never lose sight of the basic principles of emergency medicine. Knowledge and experience gained from traditional companion animal emergency medicine can be applied to reptiles. The basics are the same.

A sound history must be obtained. Pertinent questions are

What is the origin of the animal?
How long has it been in the home?
Are cage mates involved?
What type of cage setup is being used?

Box 1. Initial telephone contact

Success or failure in treatment of poisonings can stem from the initial telephone contact. Telephone personnel must establish
- The name, address, and telephone number of person calling
- Who has been poisoned? (Species, breed, age, sex, and weight)
- What toxin is involved? Try to determine the amount, concentration, and form (ie, liquid, powder, gas, or other). Are original containers listing ingredients, concentrations, potential antidotes, or manufacturer's emergency number available?
- When did the poisoning happen? How much time has elapsed since ingestion or exposure? Did the caller see it happen?
- What was the route of exposure? (Eg, ingestion, dermal, inhalation, or ocular)
- Where did it happen? (Eg, on the owner's premises?)
- How much was ingested? (Original containers allow estimation of how much was consumed and how much remains).
- What is the animal's present clinical status? (What is the animal doing? Educate the owner about the clinical signs and course of progression for that poisoning).
- Other important information:
  1. Other toxins that the animal could have been exposed to simultaneously
  2. Medications the animal is currently taking or other underlying medical conditions (eg, heart disease, kidney problems, pregnancy)
  3. Other animals or children who might have been exposed

Determine the mg/kg dosage for this exposure. Compare the amount ingested with the known therapeutic and/or toxic dose information to establish the risk for this animal. Determine a time line between exposure and onset of clinical signs for this toxin.

Determine from this information whether the animal needs to be seen and treated or can be managed conservatively at home and observed. The animal can be observed at home only if a follow-up mechanism is in place, that is, if the owner is familiar with the course of the poisoning and clinical signs and calls frequently (or is called)] with progress reports. Final recommendation to treat or observe must rest with the veterinarian.

Finally, the information gathered in the initial telephone interview allows the veterinarian to prepare for the animal's arrival, knowing what poison is involved and what clinical signs are present, and enables assembly of equipment and medications to initiate specific therapy rapidly.

Box 2. Key items in taking the toxicologic history

- Listen to the client. Avoid any bias or preconceptions.
- At the same time, observe the animal. Although one cannot always believe the client, one can believe the clinical signs of the animal.
- Identify and treat immediate life-threatening problems (eg, arrhythmias, seizures). Do not wait for confirmation of poisons involved to initiate supportive therapy.
- Identify the animal's entire home environment. Could other poisons or other animals or children be involved?
- Identify any current medications, underlying conditions, or pertinent previous medical history for the animal (eg, heart disease, kidney problems, pregnancy).
- History of the exposure event: how long ago, what toxin, what concentration, how much? Are any particular poisons present in the home because of the owner's occupation or hobbies?
- If possible, identify the poison (or poisons). Estimate the mg/kg dose for the animal and the possibility of a toxic or lethal exposure.
- Establish an exposure/onset of clinical signs time line. Is the animal getting better, deteriorating, or showing no signs?
- Establish a minimum database.
- Treat the patient, not the poison.

What heat and light sources are used? (How long a photo period is employed, what type of warming system is used and over what temperature range?).

Because the majority of reptile emergencies are secondary to inappropriate husbandry or poor diet, find out how often the animal is being fed and watered, with what diet, and how often and with what products is the cage and environment are being cleaned. This pattern of questioning can help the reptile practitioner focus most closely on the cause of the problem.

A thorough physical examination is performed next. Heart rate, respiration, hydration status, neurologic condition, and mentation are all critical cues both to diagnosis and prognosis, but history taking, physical examination, and critical signs are only part of obtaining a successful diagnosis. Laboratory parameters also help determine what treatment choices may be necessary. One must remember to keep sight of the patient's condition, to treat the patient, not the poison; likewise, laboratory results may take days or weeks to return, so one must "treat the patient, not the lab."

Box 3. Sample toxicology history form

- Animal's name, species, breed, sex, intact/neutered
- Age, weight
- Medications presently receiving
- Other pertinent medical history
- Suspected poison involved
- Maximum amount of toxin suspected (worst-case scenario)
- Was the original container found?
- Suspected route of exposure
- When did possible exposure occur?
- When were clinical signs first noted? Describe them.
- Could other poisons be involved?
- Could other animals have been exposed?
- Describe the animal's environment (where animal is kept, how long animal was left alone, hobbies of owner, anything that might lead to poisoning)

Injured, poisoned, and seriously ill reptiles nearly always benefit from fluid administration. Because of a variety of constraints, intravenous fluid administration is not practical for most reptiles, but a variety of alternative routes are available for fluid administration. Many desert reptilian species can tolerate remarkable degrees of dehydration. Chelonians, lizards, snakes, and crocodilians may display varying signs of dehydration, but for most reptiles sunken eyes and hanging skin are consistent changes. Intraosseous, enteral, intracoelomic, and subcutaneous routes of fluid administration are legitimate alternatives if intravenous pathways are not possible.

Reptiles are ectothermic and depend on environmental heat for their body temperature. Reptilian species have their own preferred body temperatures and optimum thermal zones. For most temperate species a range of 72°F to 82°F is fairly safe. Be careful! Debilitated reptiles are too weak to move away from heat sources and may overheat or even end up with thermal burns. Use only safe heat sources, such as small heating enclosures, overhead heat lights, and under-tank heating systems. Provide a gradient of temperature in the cage. Cage thermometers must be placed prominently and monitored diligently to ensure animals are kept within a safe and healthy heating range. Do not give up. Rigorous, persistent nursing care can do much to help save severely poisoned reptiles. Diets and dietary supplements are available to help support the animals as they are recovering.

The following list of poisons, by no means complete, focuses on the most common poisonings of reptiles, their mechanism of action, and any potential treatments.

Common toxicants

Vitamin A toxicity

Vitamin A is necessary for the health of normal skin and periocular tissue. Chelonians (turtles and tortoises) are particularly sensitive to vitamin A deficiency. Turtles with hypovitaminosis typically show ocular discharge, palpebral edema and blindness, hyperkeratosis of skin and mouthparts, and aural abscesses. Patients can improve with vitamin A supplementation (2000 IU/kg every 7 days) and improved dietary management [1].

Excessive iatrogenic administration of vitamin A can cause a separate set of problems. Hypervitaminosis A can cause inappetence, full-thickness skin sloughing, secondary bacterial infection, discoloration of the skin, and extreme lethargy. Generally this occurs at doses of 10,000 IU/kg or higher given intramuscularly as a single injection. Treatment involves ceasing vitamin A administration, the use of antibiotics and fluid therapy, wound management, and nutritional support. Skin lesions may heal slowly, but animals managed supportively can recover completely.

Vitamin D toxicity

Excesses of water-soluble vitamins can be excreted into the urine, making their margin of safety very large. For fat-soluble vitamins, such as vitamin A and vitamin D, the margin of safety is not as wide. Owners, breeders, and veterinarians often oversupplement captive reptiles with disastrous results. The minimum daily requirement of most vertebrates for vitamin D is only 10 to 20 IU//kg body weight [2]. Doses of 50 to 1000 times the minimum daily requirement often are given for weeks to months. The effects can be insidious. The mechanism of action of the toxicity of vitamin D is related to the hypercalcemia it induces. This prolonged hypercalcemia causes dystrophic calcification of the gastrointestinal tissue, the kidneys, lungs, heart, blood vessels, and joints [3]. Complete removal of supplements containing vitamin D and cortisone may help control hypercalcemia, but resolution of soft tissue calcification may not be successful.

In light of the inherent calcium problems of captive reptiles, it is incumbent on veterinarians to counsel clients about proper husbandry, nutrition, and dietary requirements and to ensure that no supplements are given to animals without veterinary approval.

Vitamin B₆ (pyroxidine)

Pyroxidine (water-soluble vitamin B_6) is widely available in tablet form and is used as a supplement in humans for treatment of premenstrual syndrome, by bodybuilders, and in attention deficit disorder and hyperactivity. Clinical signs of generalized weakness and sensory neuropathy have been reported in humans and dogs. Treatment of vitamin B_6 toxicity is supportive and consists of withdrawing further administration of pyroxidine.

Antimicrobial toxicity

Antibiotics should be selected judiciously. Selection depends on experience of the clinician, empiric considerations, the type of infection present based on culture, sensitivity, and gram stains, and on the size, age, species, and condition of the reptilian patient. No antibiotic is effective for all situations. In addition, antibiotics are no substitute for good wound management, nursing care, nutrition, or husbandry.

Gentamycin

Gentamycin is an aminoglycoside antibiotic. Other aminogycosides include amikacin, tobramycin, neomycin, streptomycin, and kanamycin. Gentamycin is bactericidal and is a broad-spectrum antibiotic (except against streptococci and anaerobic bacteria) [4]. Its mechanism of action involves inhibition of bacterial protein synthesis by binding to 30S ribosomes. Gentamycin is indicated for acute serious infections, such as those caused by gram-negative bacteria. Amikacin is more consistently active against resistant strains of bacteria.

Nephrotoxicity of gentamycin in reptiles is well documented [5–8]. Patients must have adequate fluid and electrolyte balance during therapy. Ototoxicity in reptiles also has been reported. Recommended dosage for gentamycin varies from 1.5 to 2.5 mg/kg given no more frequently than every third day.

Amikacin

Amikacin also is an aminoglycoside that is bactericidal, has a broad spectrum of activity, and operates on bacteria through the same mechanism of action as gentamycin. It is indicated particularly against gram-negative organisms, where it may have greater activity than gentamycin.

As with gentamycin, nephrotoxicity is the most dose-limiting effect of amikacin. Patients must be maintained in fluid and electrolyte balance during therapy. Ototoxicity also has been reported. If used together with anesthetic agents, aminoglycosides may show neuromuscular blockade. Dosages for amikacin range from 2.25 to 5 mg/kg given no more frequently than every third day.

Chloramphenicol

Chloramphenicol is an antibacterial agent with a broad spectrum of activity against gram-positive bacteria, gram-negative bacteria, and *Rickettsia*. It acts by inhibiting bacterial protein synthesis by binding with ribosomes.

The major toxicity of chloramphenicol is hematologic [9]. In all vertebrates studied, it produces direct, dose-dependent bone marrow depression resulting in reductions in red blood cells, white blood cells, and platelets. This manifestation is aggravated by inappropriate doses, extended treatments, and repeated use of the drug. Treatment of chloramphenicol intoxication is supportive and may require blood transfusions. The drug also has been reported to be appetite suppressive. Like gentamycin, chloramphenicol is being used less frequently as safer antibiotics appear. The recommended dosage for chloramphenicol is 50 mg/kg administered once daily or every other day.

Enrofloxacin

Enrofloxacin is a fluoroquinolone antibacterial drug. It is bactericidal with a broad spectrum of activity. Its mechanism of action involves inhibition of DNA gyrase, then inhibiting both DNA and RNA synthesis [4]. Sensitive bacteria include *Staphylococcus, Escherichia coli, Proteus, Klebsiella,* and *Pasteurella. Pseudomonas* is moderately susceptible but requires higher doses. In most species studied, enrofloxacin is metabolized to ciprofloxacin. Damage to cartilage has been seen in growing animals treated with fluoroquinolones. Doses of enrofloxacin range from 2.5 to 5 mg/kg. There are other choices of antibiotics for use in reptiles, based on Gram staining, culture and sensitivity, and age of animal.

Metronidazole

Metronidazole is used as an antibacterial, an antiprotozoal, an antiparasitic, and an appetite stimulant in reptiles. It is formulated as a suspension, as an injectable liquid, and as tablets.

The activity of metronidazole is specific for anaerobic bacteria and protozoa, and particularly for *Giardia* organisms. Metronidazole disrupts DNA in target microbes through reaction with intracellular metabolites [10].

The most severe side effect of metronidazole is dose-related central nervous system (CNS) toxicity. High doses can cause ataxia, inability to walk, nystagmus, opisthotonos, tremors of the lumbar muscles and hindlimbs, seizures, and death [11,12]. Treatment is symptomatic and supportive.

Metronidazole has been recommended for a variety of conditions in reptiles. When this drug is used, particular care must be taken regarding dose, duration, and size of the animal.

Antifungal toxicity

A variety of fungal infections have been documented in reptiles. Ranging from dermatophytes to systematic mycotic infections, these conditions are treated with a variety of antifungal medications. Because of the small size of the reptilian patient, the mechanism of action of these drugs, and idiosyncrasies of reptilian physiology, treatment with antifungals can lead to serious intoxications.

Amphotericin B

Amphotericin B is a macrolide-class antibiotic unrelated to erythromycin. This antifungal inhibits ergosterol synthesis [13]. Ergosterol is a component of the cell membrane unique to fungal organisms. Amphotericin is a potent nephrotoxin [14]. It produces signs of renal toxicity in 80% of patients that receive it. Its action causes renal vasoconstriction, reduces glomerular filtration rate, and has direct toxic effects on the membranes of the renal tubule cells. Through these mechanisms, amphotericin B causes acute tubular necrosis. Hypokalemia develops in almost 35% of human patients treated with amphotericin, which is sufficient to warrant potassium supplementation.

Clinical signs mimic acute renal failure, with anorexia, lethargy, weight loss, and other signs. Elevated blood urea nitrogen and creatinine levels with decreased potassium and sodium levels are seen commonly in mammals but may not be clinically relevant in reptiles [15].

Treatment includes discontinuing the drug, aggressive fluid therapy to prevent further kidney damage, and diminishing renal effects with sodium chloride–containing fluids. Treatment with mannitol may help increase the elimination of amphotericin B.

Prognosis after amphotericin B toxicity depends on the severity of the renal damage. Amphotericin B still is listed as a treatment for aspergillosis in reptiles (1 mg/kg intracoelomically once daily for 2 to 4 weeks) [16]. Safer drugs may be available. A new, less toxic formulation of amphotericin B is available for humans and soon may be available for veterinary use. Amphotericin B should not be used in animals that already have renal disease.

Griseofulvin

Griseofulvin antifungal works by inhibiting fungal spindle activity and leads to distorted, weakened fungal hyphae [17]. It also has been shown to cause bone marrow suppression in mammals, although the mechanism of this action is unknown.

Anorexia, lethargy, diarrhea, and anemia have been reported in intoxicated animals. In reptiles the recommended dosage for fungal dermatitis is 20 to 40 mg/kg given orally every third day for five treatments. It is available as a tablet and as a topical ointment.

Treatment includes discontinuing the drug and treating the patient supportively. There is no specific antidote. Griseofulvin has been shown to be teratogenic in pregnant animals of many species. Topical treatments can be removed with tepid water and gentle hand soap. Antifungal overdoses can be best avoided by preventing fungal infection through good husbandry.

Imidazoles (ketoconazole) and triazoles (fluconazole and itraconazole)

Ketoconazole, fluconazole, and itraconazole inhibit fungal replication by interfering with ergosterol synthesis. Ketoconazole also has direct effects on the fungal membrane. The liver metabolizes these fungistatic drugs. Itraconazole is more potent than ketoconazole and is better tolerated by patients.

Clinical signs of intoxication include anorexia, lethargy, weight loss, and diarrhea. Elevated liver enzymes may be present in intoxicated animals.

Dosages recommended for reptiles are 2 to 5 mg/kg orally daily for 5 days for fluconazole, 25 mg/kg given orally daily for 3 weeks for ketoconazole, and 23.5 mg/kg orally once daily for itraconazole [7]. There seems to be little problem with miconazole preparation applied topically [18].

There is no specific antidote for toxicity by these antifungals. Treatment involves stopping the drug, decontaminating any topical material remaining, and supportive therapy (fluids, warmth). For ketoconazole, treatment includes countering the hepatoxicity. Mild intoxications usually improve with simple cessation of the drug.

The safest, most effective drugs must be selected for use in treating fungal infections in reptiles, and the choice must reflect the severity of the infection, the size of the animal, and the condition of the animal before treatment. Doses must be checked meticulously, particularly for topical agents and dips to be used on reptiles. Finally, reptiles must never be left alone in any bath or medicated dip.

Organophosphates and carbamates

Organophosphates are the most commonly used insecticides worldwide. In the United Stated alone, 250 million pounds of organophosphates are used annually at a production cost of $2.4 billion [19]. They are found in agriculture, in the home, and on or around various domestic animals. Some organophosphates are meant to remain on the surfaces to which they are applied, and others are absorbed and become systemic in animals. They are the active ingredients in a long list of products. For animal use as insecticides, they are formulated as dips, sprays, topical medications, systemic parasitic agents, and flea collars. This group of insecticides includes chlorpyrifos (Dursban), dichlorvos, diazinon, cythioate (Proban), fenthion (ProSpot), malathion, ronnel, parathion, metrifonate, and Vapona. Their cousins, the carbamates include aldicarb, carbaryl (Sevin), bendiocarb, methiocarb, propoxur, and carbofuran. As newer, safer insecticides are marketed, these two groups are involved in fewer accidental poisonings, but they still account for a large number of intoxications.

Organophosphates and carbamates interfere with metabolism and breakdown of acetylcholine at synaptic junctions [20]. Acetylcholinesterase is the enzyme responsible for breaking down the neurotransmitter at these sites. Acetylcholinesterase is inhibited by organophosphates and carbamates at these cholinergic sites. As a result, acetylcholine accumulates at the synapses, first exciting and then paralyzing transmission in these synapses, leading to the characteristic "nerve gas" signs associated with organophosphate toxicity [21]. This inhibition of the synapse is irreversible with organophosphates but is reversible with carbamates. Organophosphates are readily absorbed by all routes: dermal, respiratory, gastrointestinal, and conjunctival. Overdose with organophosphates may happen more readily if they are given together with imidothiazoles, such as levamisole.

Clinical signs seen in reptiles include salivation, ataxia, muscle fascicula-tions, inability to right themselves, coma, and respiratory arrest. Death results from massive respiratory secretions, bronchiolar constriction, and effects on the respiratory centers in the medulla leading to the cessation of breathing.

Animals with dermal exposure should be washed with a mild dishwashing detergent and copious amounts of water. Animals should be dried after rins-ing to prevent further uptake of the insecticide. The need for fluid therapy to counter dehydration and electrolyte imbalances should be considered. The specific physiologic antidote, the muscarinic antagonist atropine, should be given (0.4 mg/kg intramuscularly). This agent should help with saliva-tion, bronchospasm, and dyspnea. Diazepam may be given as needed for seizures. Use of antihistamines to treat insecticide poisonings is controver-sial and may not be particularly effective. The prognosis depends on the dose, duration of exposure, and size of the animal. Therapies that are both more effective and safer than organophosphates and carbamates exist for treatment of parasites in captive reptiles. These therapeutic regimens are outlined in detail elsewhere in various sources dealing with reptilian parasitology.

Pyrethrins and pyrethroids

Pyrethrin is the oldest used botanical insecticide. It is made from the dried and ground flowers of *Chrysanthemum cinerariifolium*. Pyrethroids are syn-thetic derivatives of pyrethrin and are widely available. Pyrethroid insecti-cides have enhanced stability, potency, and half-life compared with the parent molecule. A variety of dilute pyrethrin- and pyrethroid-containing sprays have been recommended for reptiles.

Pyrethrins and pyrethroids have the same mechanism of action. These molecules affect parasites by altering the activity of the sodium ion channels of nerves. These poisons prolong the period of sodium conductance and increase the length of the depolarizing action potential [22], resulting in repetitive nerve firing and death. With the right conditions or at higher doses, these compounds can intoxicate exposed animals. Because of the potential for transcutaneous absorption, pyrethrin and pyrethroid sprays must be thoroughly rinsed from the animal immediately after their applica-tion. Rinsing with lukewarm water usually is sufficient.

Like ivermectin, organophosphates, and carbamates, pyrethrins and py-rethroids never should be given concurrently with cholinesterase-inhibiting compounds.

Clinical signs have been reported for pyrethrins and pyrethroids, partic-ularly with the use of sprays that also contain insect growth regulators (eg, methoprene). Signs can develop in animals within 15 minutes of application and include salivation, ataxia, inability to right themselves, and muscle fas-ciculations [23]. Idiosyncratic reactions to pyrethrins can happen at much lower doses than expected. A small percentage of animals seem to be extremely sensitive to pyrethrins and pyrethroids.

If caught early enough, treatment for pyrethrin and pyrethroid toxicity involves dermal decontamination (bathing in copious amounts of water), isotonic fluids, and diazepam for seizures. Care must be taken to keep pyrethrin and pyrethroid sprays away from the reptile's eyes and mouth to prevent intoxication. The prognosis depends on the strength of the agent used, the duration of the exposure, and the size of the animal involved. Animals do best when treated early.

A variety of pyrethrins and pyrethroids have been recommended for use against reptile parasites. If used prudently, these agents are safe and effective. Animals sometimes are saturated with the spray. As soon as the parasiticide is applied, it should be rinsed off. Gently running lukewarm tap water should be used to wash off the insecticide. This very brief exposure is enough to kill the parasites. To prevent absorption and systemic toxicity in host animals, pyrethrin and pyrethroid sprays should not be left on. In smaller animals that have larger surface-to-volume ratios, most sprays should be diluted to the smallest effective dose to prevent accidental intoxication from transcutaneous absorption.

Ivermectin

Ivermectin is an antiparasitic from a family of chemicals called "avermectins." These are macrocyclic lactones made from the fermentation broth of the fungus *Streptomyces avermitilis* [24]. The macrolide ivermectin is available as an injectable, a spray, and an oral formulation. It has activity against a variety of parasites including nematodes, arthropods, and arachnids.

Avermectins work by potentiating the effects of the inhibitory neurotransmitter, γ-aminobutyric acid (GABA). They stimulate release of GABA by presynaptic sites and increase GABA binding to postsynaptic receptors, causing neuromuscular blockage. Avermectins also open chloride channels in membranes of the nervous system and further depress neuronal function. These actions cause paralysis and death of susceptible parasites. Ivermectin is absorbed systemically by host tissue. When parasites bite the host, they absorb the ivermectin. Ivermectin is active against intestinal parasites, mites, microfilaria, and developing larva. Concurrent treatment with diazepam, which also works through GABA potentiation, may heighten deleterious effects.

Ivermectin can cause depression, paralysis, coma, and death in chelonians [25]. Species susceptible to ivermectin toxicosis may have a blood–brain barrier more permeable than in nonsensitive species. This greater permeability may result from p-glycoprotein mutation in membranes of the CNS. Another theory postulates the existence of a specific protein receptor present only in the brains of ivermectin-sensitive species, but this possibility has not yet been demonstrated. Ivermectin toxicity also has been reported in several species of lizards and snakes [26]. Ball pythons (*Phython regius*), in particular, may show mild neurologic signs when treated. If there is any question regarding safety, it may be more prudent to use ivermectin only as a topical.

There is no known antidote or physiologic antagonist for ivermectin. Treatment is supportive and should include decontaminating any topical sprays with soap and water, providing fluid therapy, nutritional support, monitoring electrolytes, and respiratory support. Recovery may take days to weeks. One debilitated tortoise recovered fully after 6 weeks. The authors have seen two box turtles recover completely in 4 weeks.

Ivermectin and related compounds never should be given to chelonians, pregnant animals, or neonatal individuals. Also, for particularly tiny species, other therapies should be investigated. If there is any question, ivermectin should be used only as a topical, or an alternative should be found.

Fenbendazole

Fenbendazole is a benzimidazole type of antiparasitic drug [4]. It is safe and effective against many helminth parasites in animals. Fenbendazole inhibits glucose uptake in the parasites. Because of its wide range of activity, its high degree of efficacy, and its broad margin of safety, veterinarians frequently prescribe this anthelmintic. Fenbendazole has a good margin of safety and is reported to be well tolerated, even at six times the recommended dosage and three times the recommended duration. It has been used extensively as an anthelmintic therapy in reptiles at oral dosages of 50 to 100 mg/kg once (repeated in 2 weeks) or 50 mg/kg every 24 hours for 3 to 5 days [27,28].

Toxic effects have been reported in birds, rats, cats, and dogs [29–33]. Recently, evidence of fenbendazole overdose has been reported in individuals of a small snake species given an exceedingly large dose of the drug. Four adult Fea's vipers (*Azemiops feae*) died after being administered single doses of fenbendazole ranging from 428 mg/kg to 1064 mg/kg [34]. Necropsy findings were suggestive of intestinal changes consistent with fenbendazole toxicity. Fenbendazole is regarded as a safe anthelmintic drug at recommended therapeutic doses.

Chlorhexidine toxicity

Soaking living animals in any solution can be potentially life threatening. Recently, turtles soaked for 1 hour in chlorhexidine scrub were shown to become intoxicated [35]. Cutaneous absorption of the solution and possible oral ingestion of these soaks have been postulated as the causes of the problem. Before using any substances as soak, review the literature for preferred usage, dose, and duration of the soak. Affected animals should be removed from the soak, rinsed, and supported with warmth and fluids. Remember never to leave any reptile unattended in a bath. Animals can drown much faster than anticipated. Also, particular attention must be paid to the depth of fluids in which reptiles are bathed and soaked.

Bleach

Various hypochlorite bleach solutions can be found in most households. Typically, these are 3% to 6% hypochlorite solutions in water [36]. Bleaches are moderately irritating. If contact with skin is prolonged, the damage is worsened. Bleaches can be very effective in treating cage parasites of reptiles but never should be applied to live animals. Bleach can cause alkali burns if splashed in the eyes of lizards and turtles. Immediate irrigation of the eye with copious amounts of water minimizes the damage done by the bleach. Skin exposed to bleach should be washed with a mild soap and lukewarm water. Animals should be kept out of recently bleached cages for a minimum of 24 hours to prevent respiratory tract irritation. Cages should be allowed to air out, and residual disinfectant should be removed by wiping with a clean cloth or towel.

Zinc toxicosis

Zinc is an essential trace element. It is necessary for the synthesis of more than 200 enzymes required for cell division, growth, and gene expression. Chronic zinc deficiency from improper diet is seen more commonly than acute zinc poisoning from excessive zinc intake. Zinc toxicosis may result from overzealous administration of supplements, ingestion of galvanized metal objects, zinc oxide ointment, or from ingestion of pennies. Before 1982 US pennies were more than 90% copper; since that time they are 97% zinc. The authors have seen two iguanas and one snake with gastrointestinal tracts full of pennies demonstrating signs of zinc toxicity.

The precise mechanism of action of zinc toxicosis is not known, but the red blood cells, kidney, pancreas, and liver are affected most. Intravascular hemolysis is the most consistently seen abnormality. It is thought that zinc causes oxidative damage that leads to lysis of the red blood cell membrane, in turn leading to anemia [37].

Clinical signs of zinc toxicosis depend on the amount and form of the zinc ingested. Signs are delayed if coins are the source of the zinc. As few as one or two pennies can cause toxicity. First, the animal may be anorexic and lethargic, and the zinc ingestion may mimic gastrointestinal enteritis. This manifestation is followed by intravascular hemolysis, hemoglobinemia, yellow discoloration of the skin and mucous membranes, and weight loss. Coins may be detected by palpation, but in larger animals radiographs may be necessary to reveal the pennies. Elevated zinc levels can be confirmed on a serum sample antemortem and in liver, kidney, and pancreas samples postmortem.

Treatment consists of removing the zinc-containing foreign object. Surgery may be required, but the authors have been very fortunate with removal of the coins via endoscopy. Additional supportive therapy involves fluid treatment to maintain hydration, possible blood transfusion to control anemia, and, in severe cases, use of a zinc chelator (ethylenediaminetetraacetic acid, penicillamine).

Prognosis depends on the amount of zinc ingested, the duration of the toxic exposure, and the severity of the resulting anemia. Reptiles must be kept in environments free of potential sources of zinc ingestion.

Smoke inhalation

Dangerous fires are still a daily occurrence in the new millennium. In the continental United States alone, a fire department responds to a fire call every 17 seconds [38]. Depending on the source, it is estimated that 50% to 80% of fire deaths result directly from smoke inhalation rather than from burns or trauma.

When compared with the rest of the world, the United States has one of the highest death rates caused by fire. This finding may be attributable to the wider use of synthetic materials for building and furnishings. These synthetic substances generally produce much more toxic combustion substances. In addition, the nature of buildings, with more high rises, skyscrapers, and multifloor dwellings, makes it much harder to escape from the effects of a disastrous fire and much harder to quench these fires once started.

A toxic combustion product (ie, smoke) exerts its poisonous effects by filling enclosed vital airways with gases other than oxygen and by inducing local chemical reactions in the respiratory tract. Chemical asphyxiants elicit toxic changes in tissue distant from the lung. Water solubility of toxic inhalants is the most important factor in determining the level of injury. Injury from water-soluble molecules occurs in the upper airways. Chemical toxicants with low water solubility reach the lungs, where they then exert damaging effects. In addition, the duration of exposure, the concentration of the combustion products, and the particle size of the toxin all contribute to the overall severity of the injury. Pathologic changes in the lungs and respiratory tissues may progress over hours to days.

In the authors' practice, several captive reptiles have been brought in after being exposed to the damaging smoke of house fires. Two young Ball pythons arrived after a particularly aggressive apartment fire. Direct laryngoscopy of the animals revealed the accumulation of soot and carbonaceous debris, copious secretions, and edematous laryngeal tissue. Both snakes were in severe respiratory compromise. Their breathing was weak and rapid, and the airways became increasingly edematous. The animals were treated by intubating and administering 100% oxygen, supportive fluids, and antibiotics. Despite aggressive efforts, the smaller snake continued to deteriorate and died. After 2 days of therapy, the larger snake survived. A box turtle was presented after a private residential fire. The reptile displayed no burns, was nonresponsive, and never regained consciousness despite the authors' efforts, which included supplemental oxygen, fluid therapy, antibiotics, and suctioning of airways. The turtle died roughly 2 hours after exposure. Effective management of smoke inhalation must include establishing airway patency, administration of supplemental oxygen, frequent airway suctioning and removal of both debris and secretions, and cardiovascular support. Early intubation often is more beneficial than watching for decompensation.

The management of animals suffering from smoke inhalation is labor intensive but may result in successful outcomes if animals are managed early and aggressively.

Rodenticides

Each year rodents destroy crops in the field, eat food in storage, serve as vectors for human diseases, bite people, and cause material damage by gnawing. As a result, a variety of rodenticides are employed ubiquitously in an attempt to control populations of these animals. These substances prove to be nearly as dangerous to humans and nontarget species as they are to rodents. Rodenticide intoxication has been documented in a variety of species, reptiles included. It is certainly worth the effort for the owner to bring in the original container housing the poison so that active ingredients can be positively identified and appropriate treatment can be initiated.

Anticoagulants

The long-acting anticoagulants are responsible for 80% of rodenticide poisonings in humans and animals in the United States [38]. The long-acting agents have the same mechanism of action as warfarin, but they are more potent, and their half-life is longer. Unlike older rodenticides, they are effective in single or very limited feedings. They act by decreasing the activity of the vitamin K–dependent blood-clotting factors (II, VII, IX, and X). When clotting factors are sufficiently reduced, bleeding occurs. The most common and most toxic second-generation anticoagulants in use are brodifacum and bromadiolone.

Clinical signs depend on the site and extent of hemorrhage. The majority of intoxicated animals show anorexia, weakness, and lethargy [39]. The most common clinical sign is dyspnea. Typically animals bleed into body cavities, abdomen, thorax, and joints. Most of these poisons are packaged as molasses-soaked grain laced with the anticoagulants. These various plant materials can attract herbivorous or omnivorous reptiles. Newer formulations of the baits are dyed turquoise.

The authors have seen one iguana and one box turtle intoxicated by the ingestion of anticoagulant bait. Baseline determinations of buccal mucosal bleeding time (BMBT) or one-stage prothrombin time (PT) are helpful in animals suspected of consuming anticoagulant poisons. One antidote for anticoagulant poisoning, vitamin K_1, should be administered in animals if the BMBT or PT is increased. Although PT or BMBT are not established for all reptile species, the authors think that measuring BMBT is useful and relevant in reptiles. The daily dose recommendation for vitamin K_1 is 2.5 mg/kg. Therapy with this antidote must be maintained until toxic amounts of the poison no longer are present in the animal. Length of treatment depends on the dose and type of the anticoagulant ingested but may be as long as 3 to 4 weeks. A PT or BMBT test should be run 48 hours after cessation of vitamin K_1 treatment. If clotting time is normal, therapy is discontinued. If the clotting time is increased, therapy is continued for another week. Vitamin K_1 treatment can be given by subcutaneous injection or orally. Intravenous injections have a high incidence of anaphylactic reaction. Other treatment options include possible oxygen support and plasma transfusions.

Bromethalin

Bromethalin is one of the newer rodenticides. It is formulated in baits of pelleted grain and may be dyed green or turquoise. Bromethalin is a neurotoxin, but because of its name it can be confused with the long-acting anticoagulants bromadiolone and brodifacoum. Clients should be encouraged to bring in original containers to obtain valuable label information concerning ingredients.

The mechanism of action of bromethalin is the uncoupling of oxidative phosphorylation. The brain is the primary target for bromethalin because of its unique dependence on oxidative phosphorylation. The drug causes brain electrolyte disturbances and results in the development of cerebral edema [40].

Clinical signs include hindlimb paralysis, abnormal postures, fine muscle tremors, and seizures. Severely poisoned animals are comatose. Clinical signs are usually seen within 24 hours of ingestion.

Bromethalin is a nonselective vertebrate poison. No antidote exists, and treatment is directed initially at reducing gastrointestinal absorption and providing supportive care. Treatment also must aim at controlling cerebral edema seen in severe poisonings. Administration of dexamethasone and mannitol has been recommended to control bromethalin-induced cerebral edema. Unfortunately these diuretic agents are not very effective in controlling bromethalin-poisoned animals. Animals showing severe signs, such as seizures, paralysis, or coma, generally have a grave prognosis.

Cholecalciferol

Cholecalciferol (vitamin D_3), a newer rodenticide, exploits rodents' extreme sensitivity to small percentage changes in the calcium balance in their blood. Cholecalciferol causes hypercalcemia through mobilization of the body's calcium stores, predominantly found in bone [41]. This dystrophic hypercalcemia results in calcification of blood vessels, organs, and soft tissue. It leads to nerve and muscle dysfunction and cardiac arrhythmias.

The rodenticide is formulated in pelleted baits of grain or seed. Accidental ingestion of human medication containing vitamin D_3 or its analogues by animals is also possible. Iatrogenic oversupplementation of vitamin D_3 to reptiles also is likewise possible.

Clinical signs include depression, weakness, and anorexia. Eventually signs of renal disease become evident as the glomerular filtration rate decreases.

Treatment usually involves corticosteroid and diuretic therapy. Corticosteroids suppress bone resorption, intestinal calcium absorption, and promote calciuresis. Prednisone (6 mg/kg) and furosemide (1 to 4 mg/kg) have been recommended [41,42]. Supportive fluids (physiologic saline) are essential. Calcitonin therapy has been recommended, but its efficacy is questionable. Pamidronate disodium (Aredia), a biphosphonate, has been recommended in dogs with 1 to 2 mg/kg given slowly (over 2 hours) [42].

Prognosis is poor when dystrophic mineralization already has occurred.

Metaldehyde

Metaldehyde is the active ingredient in most slug and snail baits. It is formulated as granules, powder, pellets, and a liquid. Protein-rich materials, such as bran or grain, usually are added to the bait to make it more attractive to snails. Unfortunately, other animals find it more palatable as a result. Metaldehyde poisoning has been reported in a wide range of species ranging from dogs to livestock. Metaldehyde intoxication is uncommon in reptiles; however, the authors did see one captive tortoise fatality after encountering the poison in a household backyard garden.

The mechanism of action of metaldehyde poisoning once was thought to be a result of the degradation of the compound to acetaldehyde. Recent studies suggest metaldehyde itself may be the agent that affects the CNS [43]. GABA levels are decreased by metaldehyde, and this decrease can lead to depression, seizures, and coma.

Clinical signs include ataxia, incoordination and locomotor signs, muscle spasms, abnormal postures, and convulsions [44]. The tortoise involved presented as comatose, nonresposive, and with the head and legs rigidly extended. Clinical signs develop within a few hours of ingestion.

There is no specific antidote for metaldehyde poisoning. Instead, animals are treated supportively. Fluids should be given and oxygen administered to counter respiratory depression. Mammals may display the "shake and bake" syndrome, are treated with diazepam or other appropriate anticonvulsants, and steps are taken to counter the hyperthermia. Prognosis generally is better if the animal survives the first 35 hours. The public is strangely unaware of the hazards of this potent poison.

Mushrooms

Confirmed mushroom toxicities are relatively rare, but the potential for such poisonings remains constant. For humans poisoned by mushrooms in the United States, the exact species is never identified in more than 95% of the cases [45,46]. Furthermore, humans known to have ingested toxic mushrooms show no symptoms more than 50% of the time. By far the most toxic North American mushrooms are members of the *Amanita* species. The next most dangerous are hallucinogenic mushrooms.

This relative rarity of mushroom poisoning, the scarcity of lethal or even serious ingestions, and the inability of most physicians and veterinarians to identify correctly the mushroom species involved complicate the successful diagnosis of such toxicities. Nevertheless, a successful strategy and treatment plan for suspected mushroom poisoning is necessary.

Veterinarians must strive to learn the toxic varieties of mushrooms in their region and their general incidence. Successful diagnosis includes gross identification of the mushroom specimen and a microscopic spore assessment ("spore-prints") by trained mycologists. Investigation and confirmation of species by such collaboration is crucial to distinguishing toxic mushrooms from those that are edible.

Captive reptiles can be exposed to mushrooms in yards and greenhouses, in household terrariums, and as additives to their diet. Owners witnessing potential toxic mushroom ingestions in small animals must be instructed to bring portions of the culprit mushroom in for identification. The authors saw one case in which a pet iguana ingested *Amanita pantherina* in a backyard. Within 30 minutes of ingestion, the approximately 10-kg lizard became lethargic and ataxic. The owners brought parts of that and other mushrooms along with the lizard.

A pantherina is found throughout the United States and usually exists singly. It has a brilliant red cap and often is photographed by naturalists because of its dramatic appearance. These mushrooms contain ibotenic acid and muscimol, its decarboxylated metabolite. Ibotenic acid is related structurally to the stimulatory transmitter agent, glutamic acid [45]. Muscimol is very similar to the neurotransmitter, GABA, and acts as a GABA agonist with typical GABA signs and manifestations.

Treatment is supportive. Most GABA manifestations respond to supportive care, and the animals completely recover. Benzodiazepines, such as diazepam, may be required for the management of seizures.

The iguana treated by the authors responded within a few hours to fluids, warmth, and tube feeding. No long-lasting effects were noted, and the animal was released after 24 hours. This case illustrates the value of owners bringing in the mushroom involved for correct identification. Veterinarians must establish solid contacts with other local health professionals, such as human toxicologists, university mycologists, and laboratories well versed in toxicologic analysis.

Plant poisonings

Some plants can produce very powerful poisons. For many years veterinary toxicology dealt largely with livestock suffering from plant poisonings. The last 20 years have seen a tremendous growth in the understanding of small animal intoxications [47]. Because many reptiles are partially or entirely herbivorous, the potential for the accidental ingestion of toxic plants is very real (Box 4). Consideration of all plants that are potentially toxic to reptiles is beyond the scope of the present discussion. This section examines the more frequently encountered plant poisonings and those commonly reported in the literature.

Heaths

Plants in the heath family (eg, azaleas, laurel, rhododendrons) are planted commonly in the United States as ornamental shrubbery. These plants contain grayanotoxins (diterpenoids) that interfere with membrane-based sodium channels [48]. The toxin is found in the stem, leaves, flowers, and nectar. Dogs and people may have bradycardia. Ingestion of small amounts can lead to gastrointestinal signs; larger amounts can cause depression, ataxia, and convulsions. No antidote exists, and treatment is supportive. The authors have seen two iguanas stricken after eating azalea, and one of the lizards subsequently died. The authors also are aware of a case in which three tortoises ingested rhododendron leaves; all three died.

Yews

Ground hemlock, Florida yew, English yew, Pacific yew, and Japanese yew are members of a group of shrubs and trees that contain taxine, a cardiotoxic

---

Box 4. Factors affecting the potential toxicity of poisonous plants

Geographic and seasonal variables
- Plants known to be poisonous in one part of the world may not be as toxic in other areas.
- The season also may affect toxicity of plants.

Plant part ingested
- Not all parts of poisonous plants are always toxic.
- Tomatoes are a very edible fruit, but the stems and leaves contain toxic alkaloids.
- Apples, peaches, and apricots possess cyanide-containing seeds, although the fruit itself is edible.

Absorbability of toxins
- In apples, peaches, apricots: cyanide is not released unless seeds are broken.
- Castor bean: poison (ricin) is not released unless seeds are chewed.

Species ingesting the plant
- To a large degree, poisonous plant intoxication depends directly on which species has done the ingesting.

alkaloid. This substance is a sodium-channel blocker that can cause both cardiac and neurologic toxicity [49]. The bark, leaves, and seeds of these ornamental shrubs are poisonous, but the red fruit surrounding the seeds are not. No antidote exists. Poisonings have been reported in livestock, dogs, and caged birds.

Lilies

Easter lily, tiger lily, day lily, Japanese show lily, and Asiatic lily are known to be poisonous to cats by causing renal toxicosis [50]. All parts of the plant are poisonous. In addition, lily of the valley contains a potent cardiac glycoside. In the authors' experience, toxic plant ingestion by reptiles is possible; animals in captivity are exposed to all sorts of plants they would not encounter in their native environments. The authors have administered activated charcoal to an iguana that ingested Easter lilies. In general, treatment is supportive.

Fruit seeds

The seed of apples, apricots, cherries, peaches, plums, and the jetberry bush contain cyanogenic glycosides. The seeds are dangerous if the seed capsule is broken. In humans, as few as 5 to 25 broken seeds can cause cyanide toxicosis [51]. Cyanide disrupts the ability of cells to use oxidative phosphorylation by poisoning mitochondria. The net effect is tissue hypoxia. The onset of clinical signs may be very rapid, and death can occur suddenly. Treatment for cyanide toxicosis, which often is unsuccessful, includes 100% oxygen administration, supplemental fluids, and perhaps sodium nitrite or sodium thiosulfate. Attention must be given to what captive reptiles are eating, being fed, or are able to come into contact with.

Avocado

Avocado (*Persea americana*) has been shown to be toxic to rabbits, mice, and caged birds [52]. All parts of the plant growing above ground are toxic. Persin, a compound isolated from the leaves, is believed to be the toxin responsible for avocado toxicity. Intoxicated mammals display cardiac arrhythmias, necrosis of the myocardium, and acute death. Caged birds show respiratory distress. Until more is known about the nature of avocado poisoning, avocados should not be included in the diet of herbivorous captive reptiles.

Ricin (castor bean intoxication)

Castor bean plants contain ricin, a potent toxin in that inhibits protein synthesis. The poison is present in the whole plant but is most concentrated in the seed [53]. Chewing or breaking the seed coat is necessary before intoxication can take place. For mice, rats, rabbits, and dogs, only one seed can be fatal. In dogs clinical signs involve the gastrointestinal tract but can lead to kidney failure and convulsions. No known antidote is available. All ingestions of castor beans should be taken seriously because of the high toxicity of ricin, but seed coats are not always chewed or broken when animals ingest seeds.

Cycad (sago) palms

Sago palms are used as houseplants and occur naturally in tropical and subtropical regions. All parts of the plant are toxic. The nuts (seeds) are most toxic and are produced only by female plants. The toxins induce gastrointestinal and hepatic signs (cycasin) neurologic signs (B-methyla-mino-L-alanine); an unknown toxin causes additional neurologic signs [54]. Gastrointestinal signs generally appear within 24 hours of ingestion. No antidote exists, and treatment is supportive. Clients should be encouraged to bring in the chewed plant to help identify the species. It is astonishing how many people do not know the type of plants they have in their home or yard.

Holly, mistletoe, and poinsettia

During the holiday season, several potentially toxic plants are brought into the home. Although their toxicity is exaggerated, reptiles may blunder into them. This section gives an overview of the most common holiday plants.

Mistletoes (*Phoradendron* species) are evergreen parasitic plants that grow on trees. Human exposures usually involve the berries, either eaten by small children or brewed into tea [55]. Attempts to reproduce clinical signs in animals have been unsuccessful. In humans the most common clinical signs are gastrointestinal. No antidote is available, and treatment is supportive.

Holly (*Ilex* species) includes the English or Christmas holly, American or white holly, and winterberry. Berries contain the saponin, ilicin, which is a potent gastrointestinal irritant [55]. In humans and companion mammalian species, the most common sign is upset of the digestive tract. No antidote exists, and treatment is supportive.

Poinsettia (*Euphorbia pulcherrima*) possesses a milky sap rich in diterpenoids. These molecules are fairly irritating to the skin, mucous membranes, and gastrointestinal tract. Reports of toxicity stem from a single account [55]. Poisoning is rare, and treatment is supportive.

Cardiac glycosides

Several plants, including oleander (*Nerium oleander*), foxglove (*Digitalis purpurea*), and lily of the valley (*Convallaria majalis*), contain cardiac glycosides [56]. All parts of the oleander leaf are poisonous; a single well-chewed leaf has been reported to be lethal. Foxglove leaves and seeds are toxic. Lily of the valley poisoning occurs from ingestion of the leaves, flowers, or roots. The cardiac glycosides are gastrointestinal irritants, may be responsible for a variety of cardiac arrhythmias (eg, irregular pulse, bradycardia, rapid thready pulse, ventricular fibrillation), and can be fatal. With plant ingestions, the exact amount of toxin involved is never known.

Ivy

Ivy (*Hedera* species) is used in greenhouses, as a houseplant, and as a ground cover. English ivy, Irish ivy, Persian ivy, Atlantic ivy, and others are all potentially toxic. These plants, particularly the berries, contain terpenoids. These molecules can cause salivation, gastrointestinal irritation, and diarrhea. Most ingestions are not serious, and treatment is supportive.

Nicotine

Tobacco products including pipe tobacco, cigarettes, cigars, chewing tobacco, and snuff contain the alkaloid nicotine. Nicotine is a stimulant of the central nervous and cardiovascular systems. It stimulates sympathetic ganglia and increases heart rate and blood pressure [57]. High-dose exposures can cause paralysis of the chest muscles and lead to respiratory compromise and cardiac arrest. Cigarettes contain an average 5 to 25 mg of nicotine depending on the brand. Cigars have four to five times the nicotine content of cigarettes. Chewing tobacco is even more palatable to animals because of added flavors (eg, honey, sugar, molasses, cinnamon, licorice, various syrups). Aids to stop smoking also can be a source of accidental nicotine ingestion. Nicotine patches usually contain between 7 and 25 mg, and nicotine gum contains 2 to 4 mg per piece [58]. Some garden spray insecticides (eg, Black Leaf 40) contain 40% nicotine.

Captive reptiles may ingest cigar and cigarette butts, pipe tobacco, chewing tobacco, or nicotine patches and gums. The authors have seen one tortoise and one iguana die after eating cigarette butts. Clinical signs of high-dose nicotine intoxication include excitement followed by depression, diarrhea, seizures, coma, and respiratory or cardiac arrest. There is no known antidote. Treatment includes frequent monitoring of heart rate, and animals may benefit from fluid therapy and oxygen administration. Prognosis is poor for high-dose intoxications. As few as two cigarettes have been shown to cause lethal poisonings. No data exist for secondary cigarette smoke intoxication, but an association between chronic respiratory conditions in captive reptiles and households with one or more smokers has been suspected.

Oak poisoning

Oak trees are found almost worldwide. Acorns, buds, twigs, and leaves have been implicated in poisonings, but most incidents of intoxication involve either immature leaves in the spring or freshly fallen acorns in the spring.

Toxicosis from oak is produced by high concentrations of tannic acid and its metabolites, gallic acid, and pyrogallol [59]. Ingestion of toxic amounts of oak has been shown to cause ulcerative lesions in the upper and lower gastrointestinal tract, liver lesions, and necrosis of proximal renal tubular epithelial cells.

A fatal episode of oak intoxication has been reported in a tortoise. An African spurred tortoise (*Geochelone sulcata*) was found dead in an outdoor enclosure possessing numerous oaks hanging over and into the area [60]. Necropsy of the tortoise revealed a markedly distended stomach with partially digested oak leaves. Extensive necrosis was found in the oral cavity, esophagus, stomach, and kidneys. The proximal renal tubules showed 45% necrosis.

Grapes and raisins

Although grapes and raisins have been reported to be toxic to some dogs, no signs of grape or raisin toxicosis have been reported as yet in reptiles. Many omnivorous and herbivorous lizards and chelonians routinely eat grapes.

Marijuana

Marijuana continues to be by far the most widely used illicit drug in the United States [61]. *Cannabis sativa* has been used for centuries for its hemp fiber, as rope, and for its psychoactive resins. Totally or partially herbivorous captive reptiles may encounter growing marijuana plants or ingest dried stems, leaves, and flowers.

The main active ingredient of marijuana is tetrahydrocannabinol (THC) [62]. The highest concentration of this psychoactive constituent is found in the leaves and the flowering tops of plants. Hashish is the dried resin of flower tops. The precise mechanism of action of THC is unknown, but the psychoactive effects of this drug are thought to stem from a number of sites within the CNS, including cholinergic, dopaminergic, serotoninergic, noradrenergic, and GABA receptors. Ingested marijuana induces clinical signs much more slowly than the inhaled smoke; however, the effects of ingested THC last much longer.

Clinical signs after ingestion of marijuana include mydriasis, weakness, ataxia, bradycardia, hypothermia, and stupor. The extent of clinical signs following marijuana ingestion is almost totally dose related.

Treatment for marijuana ingestion is primarily supportive and symptomatic. Marijuana intoxications are rarely fatal because of the wide margin of safety of THC. Activated charcoal administration is recommended to decrease enterohepatic recirculation. Despite its relative safety margin, recovery following ingestion may be prolonged and take up to 3 to 4 days. Fluids and monitoring body temperature may be beneficial.

The authors have seen two reptiles that ingested fairly large amounts of marijuana. A 10-pound Sulcata tortoise showed no effects after eating four marijuana cigarettes, but a 6-pound male green iguana was stuporous after eating into a "baggie" of marijuana. Both animals recovered completely.

Undoubtedly, reptiles have blundered across other illicit drugs. Captive reptiles given free range in the house also may encounter various over-the-counter drugs kept on nightstands, kitchen counters, or bathroom shelves. For their own safety, captive animals should be confined, and all medications should be kept in their original containers in child- and animal-proof cabinets.

Venomous and poisonous animals

Snake envenomation

Snake venoms are complex mixtures of enzymatic and nonenzymatic proteins [63]. Derived from modified salivary glands, snake venoms immobilize prey and predigest their tissue. Hyaluronidase is present in most snake venom and works by catalyzing the cleavage of internal glycoside bonds and mucopolysaccharides. This action potentiates the activity of many of the other toxic agents. Many snake venoms contain phospholipase A, which causes hydrolytic breakdown of membrane phospholipids [64]. This molecule has cytotoxic, anticoagulant (preventing activation of clotting factors), and neurotoxic activities. Collagenase, also found in snake venom, leads to the digestion of collagen and the breaking down of connective tissue.

Snake venoms are incredibly complex diverse combinations of toxins and may vary, even between closely related species [65,66]. Many of the toxic principals in snake venom have yet to be identified precisely. Snake venom toxins usually are named either after the snake venom in which they were first identified or after their primary pharmacologic effect on the victim.

Snake venoms are approximately 90% water and, in addition to enzymatic and nonenzymatic proteins, can contain lipids, carbohydrates, and biogenic amines. The actual toxins, which compose the "killing fraction," are referred to as "venins." The entire mixture is called "venom." Neutralizing antibodies to the toxins of their own venom have been documented in the serum of many snakes, but the authors have seen fatalities in venomous snakes bitten by conspecifics. The severity of the response seems to depend on the location of the bite, the volume of venom injected, and the size of the bite recipient. The authors also, however, have seen bites by conspecifics and self-inflicted bites that were nonfatal.

Certain nonvenomous snake species that prey on other snakes (including venomous ones), such as the king snake, *Lampropeltis getulus*, also seem to have some resistance to venom [67].

Effective antivenins exist for some venomous snake venoms.

Poisonous lizards

Among the approximately 3000 species of lizards, only two species are known to be poisonous [68]: the Gila monster *Heloderma suspectum* (with two subspecies) and the Mexican beaded lizard *Heloderma horridum* (with three subspecies). Both species are found only in the Americas. Their venom is used only in defense [69].

The venom of these lizards in antigenically unrelated to snake venom [70]. The venom glands are in the lower jaw, and the venom is delivered to the gums at the base of the teeth. Delivery of the venom requires intense chewing action.

Heloderma venom consists of multiple enzymatic proteins including hyaluronidase, phospholipase, arginine hydrolase, and kallikrein-like enzymes.

Other proteins have been identified in this venom, including gilatoxin and helothermine.

Hyaluronidase acts as a spreading factor, decreases the viscosity of connective tissue, and catalyzes the cleavage of acid mucoglycosides. Arginine hydrolase causes hydrolysis of peptide linkages, and the kallikrein-like enzymes cause vasodilation, increase capillary permeability, lead to edema, and affect the contraction or relaxation of extravascular smooth muscle.

Phospholipase has been documented in many types of venom and contributes by releasing other enzymes leading to membrane destruction. It also stimulates the release of histamine, kinin, and serotonin. Gilatoxin is a neurotoxic protein. Helothermine has been shown to depress the body temperature in mice subjected to this poison [71]. Bites of these lizards in humans have been reported as very painful. Currently, no specific antivenin for venomous lizard bites is available, and treatment is supportive. Gila monsters seem to be relatively resistant to the effects of their own venom.

Amphibian toxins

Certain amphibians are poisonous and can cause intoxications. In the United States two toad species (genus *Bufo*) are the source of the majority of toad poisonings. The cane or marine toad (*Bufo marinus*) and the Colorado River toad (*Bufo alvarius*) are the two species most often implicated [72,73].

All *Bufo* species of toads have parotid glands that release toxic substances when the animals are threatened. These toxic substances are biologically active compounds, such as dopamine, norepinephrine, epinephrine, serotonin, bufotenine, bufogenin, bufotoxins, and indolealkylamines. Severe toxicosis has been seen in small animals that bite, masticate, or hold these toads in their mouths. The active compounds secreted from the toad's parotid gland are absorbed rapidly by the mucous membranes of the predator and enter the systemic circulation.

Once these compounds have entered the circulation, the greatest effects are seen on the peripheral vascular system, the CNS, and the heart. Bufotenine has pressor effects on blood vessels but may act as a hallucinogen as well. Bufogenin has digitalis-like effects [74]. It causes alterations in heart rate and rhythm. Bufotoxins are vasoconstrictors and add to the pressor effects. Indolealkylamines have activity similar to the hallucinogen LSD.

Dogs are the animals most commonly affected by amphibian parotid toxins, but cats and ferrets have been reported to be affected. Exposure in reptiles has not been documented; however, it is logical to assume predatory reptiles that include amphibians in their diet might encounter and ingest poisonous toads. No specific antidote is available, and treatment is basically supportive. Therapy includes thoroughly flushing the oral cavity with running water. Severely affected animals may require seizure intervention and medications to stabilize heart rhythms. Supportive care involving fluids may be necessary in badly debilitated animals. Many other toxicoses and conditions can lead to neuropathies, and cardiac arrhythmias can present with signs very similar to those of toad poisonings.

Firefly toxicosis

Reptile caretakers often supplement the diet of captive animals with freshly caught insects. Fireflies of the genus *Photinus* have been shown to contain steroidal pyrones (lucibufagins) that are poisonous [75–77]. Structurally the pyrones are similar to cardenolides of plants and bufodienolides of toads, both of which are well-studied toxins [78,79]. These two compounds cause nausea and vomiting at low concentrations and can be potentially cardiotoxic at higher doses. If extrapolations from mammals are correct, less than one half of a firefly could be lethal to a 100-g lizard.

Lucibufagins protect fireflies from predators [80]. Spiders, birds, and several species of lizard have been shown to avoid fireflies [81,82]. Like many lizards, bearded dragons show indiscriminate eating strategies and may ingest toxic substances. Furthermore, the bearded dragon, an Australian native, has no natural contact with *Photinus* species of fireflies and thus may exhibit no self-protective avoidance behavior.

Other lizard species have been shown to eat fireflies without lethal results. In one study both Fence Lizards (*Scleroporus undulatus*) and Skinks (*Eumeces laticep*) were fed fireflies. Both species readily attacked and ate the insects but spit them out immediately, wiping their mouths and rubbing their faces on the ground. When offered fireflies a second time (even days later), they refused to eat them and exhibited the same mouth wiping that they displayed after tasting the insects. Next, the researchers placed five to seven fireflies into live crickets. Both species of lizards ate the crickets but subsequently regurgitated all the crickets they had eaten. No lizards of either type died after eating the fireflies. This study concluded that fireflies were distasteful and could cause regurgitation and vomiting, but the ingestion of fireflies is not always lethal to all lizard species.

Keepers must be advised to feed only safe food items. Any questions should be referred to a veterinarian. Fireflies should not be fed to reptiles, nor should any insects that sequester cardenolides, such as monarch butterflies (*donaus plexippus*), queen butterflies (*Donaus gilippus*), and lygaeid bug (*Oncopeltus fasciatus*). Other lizard species and other captive reptiles may be susceptible to intoxication following firefly ingestion, and fireflies should not be offered as food [83].

Dioctyl sodium sulfosuccinate

Dioctyl sodium sulfosuccinate (DSS) is an anionic surfactant substance that traditionally has been recommended as a laxative and stool softener for a variety of vertebrates ranging from humans to rodents. DSS has been advocated for the same use in reptiles.

DSS generally regarded as a relatively safe pharmaceutical agent with a low toxicity, but reports of toxic effects exist in the literature for horses, dogs, monkeys, rats, rabbits, guinea pigs, and mice after either oral or topical administration [84–90]. Furthermore, fatalities in reptiles after oral use of DSS have been reported [91]. One study documents severe changes in gastric and esophageal mucosa in Gopher snakes (*Pituophis melanoleucus*) given oral DSS at a dosage of 250 mg/kg.

A specific dose of DSS has not been established for reptiles, but dosages for other species range from 15 to 40 mg/kg for dogs and cats to 200 mg/kg for horses [89,92]. Concentrations (dilutions) of 1:30 have been recommended for reptiles [93]. A DSS dosage of 1-5 mg/kg PO has been recommended.

The study in the gopher snakes and the several reports in various other species indicate that DSS may not be as innocuous as once popularly believed. These studies demonstrate that DSS can have adverse effects, and, in reptiles, levels greater than 250 mg/kg can cause caustic changes to epithelial surfaces. In addition, the potential for overzealous administration of DSS leading to aspiration pneumonia clearly exists in captive reptiles. Extreme care must be taken if DSS is to be used, and the use of other laxatives, stool softeners, and enhancers of gastric motility should be explored.

References

[1] Rossi JV. Dermatology. In: Mader DR, editor. Reptile medicine and surgery. Philadelphia: WB Saunders; 1996.
[2] Frye FL. Biomedical and surgical aspects of captive reptile husbandry. vol. 2. 2nd edition. Melbourne (FL): Krieger Publishing; 1991.
[3] Lewis LD, Morris JL Jr, Hand MS, et al. Small animal clinical nutrition. Topeka (KS): Mack Morris Assoc; 1987.
[4] Papich MG. Handbook of veterinary drugs. Philadelphia: WB Saunders; 2002.
[5] Montali RJ, Bush M, Smeller JM. The pathology of nephrotoxicity of gentamycin in snakes. Vet Pathol 1979;16:108–15.
[6] Bagger-Sjoback D, Wesall J. Toxic effects of gentamycin on the basilar papilla in the lizard Calotes vericolor. Acta Otolaryngol 1976;81:57.
[7] Funk RS. A formulary for lizards, snakes, and crocodilians. Vet Clin North Am Exot Pract 2000;3(1):333–58.
[8] Klingenberg RJ. Therapeutics. In: Mader DR, editor. Reptile medicine and surgery. Philadelphia: WB Saunders; 1996.
[9] Holt D, Harvey J, Hurley R. Chloramphenicol toxicity. Adverse Drug React Toxicol Rev 1993;12:83–95.
[10] Papich MG. Metronidazole. In: Papich MG, editor. Handbook of veterinary drugs. Philadelphia: WB Saunders; 2002.
[11] Bennett RA. Neurology. In: Mader DR, editor. Reptile medicine and surgery. Philadelphia: WB Saunders; 1996.
[12] Lawton MPC. Neurological disease. In: Benyon PH, editor. Manual of reptiles, British small animal veterinary association. Ames (IA): Iowa State University Press; 1992.
[13] Haddad LM, Herman SM. Antibiotics and anthelminthics. In: Haddad LM, Shannon MW, Winchester JF, editors. Clinical management of poisoning and drug overdose. Philadelphia: WB Saunders; 1998.

[14] Hoitsma AJ, et al. Drug-induced nephrotoxicity aetiology, clinical features, and management. Drug Saf 1991;6(2):131.

[15] Plumb DC. Veterinary drug handbook. 3rd edition. Ames (IA): Iowa State University Press; 1999.

[16] Bonner BB. Chelonian therapeutics. Vet Clin North Am Exotic Pract 2000;3(1):207–32.

[17] Roder JD. Antimicrobials. In: Plumlee KH, editor. Clinical veterinary toxicology. St. Louis (MO): Mosby; 2004.

[18] Scott FW, et al. Teratogenesis in cats associated with griseofulvin therapy. Teratology 1975; 11:79.

[19] Carlton FB, Simpson WM, Haddad LM. The organophosphates and other insecticides. In: Haddad LM, Shannon MW, Winchester JF, editors. Clinical management of poisoning and drug overdose. Philadelphia: WB Saunders; 1998.

[20] Blodgett DJ. Organophosphate and carbamate insecticides. In: Peterson ME, Talcott PA, editors. Small animal toxicology. Philadelphia: WB Saunders; 2001.

[21] Jamal GA. Neurological syndromes of organophosphorus compounds. Adverse Drug React Toxicol Rev 1997;16(3):133–70.

[22] Hansen SR. Pyrethrins and pyrethroids. In: Peterson ME, Talcott PA, editors. Small animal toxicology. Philadelphia: WB Saunders; 2001.

[23] Denardo D, Wozniak EJ. Understanding the snake mite and current therapies for control. Proc Assoc of Rept Amph Veterin 1997;7:137–47.

[24] Papich MG. Ivermectin. In: Papich MG, editor. Handbook of veterinary drugs. Philadelphia: WB Saunders; 2002.

[25] Teare JD, Bush M. Toxicity and efficacy of ivermectin in chelonians. J Am Vet Med Assoc 1983;183(11):1195.

[26] Wosniak EJ, et al. Ectoparasites. J Herpetol Med Surg 2000;10(3):15–21.

[27] Stein G. Reptile and amphibian formulary. In: Mader DR, editor. Reptile medicine and surgery. Philadelphia: WB Saunders; 1996.

[28] Carpenter JW, Mashima TY, Rupiper DJ. Exotic animal formulary. Philadelphia: WB Saunders; 2001.

[29] Dalvi RR. Comparative studies on the effect of fenbendazole on the liver and liver enzymes of goats, quail, and rats. Vet Res Commun 1989;13:135–9.

[30] Howard LL, et al. Benzimidazole toxicity in birds. Proceedings of the Annual Conference of the American Association of Zoo Veterinarians 1999;36.

[31] Papendick RI, et al. Suspected fenbendazole toxicity in birds. Proc Annu Conf Am Assoc Zoo Vet 1998;144–6.

[32] Shoda T, et al. Liver tumor promoting effects of fenbendazole in rats. Toxicol Pathol 1999; 27:553–62.

[33] Stokol T, et al. Development of bone marrow toxicosis after albendazole administration in a dog and a cat. J Am Vet Med Assoc 1997;210:1753–6.

[34] Alvarado TP, et al. Fenbendazole overdose in four Fea's vipers (*Azemiops feae*). Proc Assoc Rept Amph Vet 1997;35–6.

[35] Lloyd ML. Chlorhexidine toxicosis in a part of red-bellied short-necked turtles. Emudura subglosa. Bull Rept Amph Vet 1996;6(4):6–7.

[36] Mcguigan MA. Bleach, soaps, detergents, and other corrosives. In: Haddad EM, Shannon MW, Winchester JF, editors. Clinical management of poisoning and drug overdose. 3rd edition. Philadelphia: WB Saunders; 1998.

[37] Talcott PA. Zinc poisoning. In: Peterson ME, Talcott PA, editors. Small animal toxicology. Philadelphia: WB Saunders; 2001.

[38] Holstege CP, Metts BC, Kirk MA, et al. Smoke inhalation. In: Goldfrank LR, et al, editors. Toxologic emergencies. 7th edition. New York: McGraw-Hill; 2002.

[39] Murphy JM, Talcott PA. Anticoagulant rodenticides. In: Peterson ME, Talcott PA, editors. Small animal toxicology. Philadelphia: WB Saunders; 2001.

[40] Dorman DL. Bromethalin in small animal toxicology. Philadelphia: WB Saunder; 2001. p. 435–44.

[41] Rumbeiha WK. Cholecalciferol. In: Peterson ME, Talcott PA, editors. Small animal toxicology. Philadelphia: WB Saunders; 2001.

[42] Morrow CK, Volmer PA. Cholecalciferol. In: Plumlee KH, editor. Clinical veterinary toxicology. St. Louis (MO): Mosby; 2004.

[43] Puschner B. Metaldehyde. In: Peterson ME, Talcott PA, editors. Small animal toxicology. Philadelphia: WB Saunders; 2001.

[44] Gfeller RW, Messonnier SP. Metaldehyde. In: Gfeller RW, Messonnier SP. Handbook of small animal toxicology and poisonings. St. Louise (MO): Mosby; 2004.

[45] Goldfrank LR. Mushrooms. In: Goldfrank LR, et al, editors. Goldfrank's toxicologic emergencies. 7th edition. New York: McGraw-Hill; 2002.

[46] Benjamin DR. Mushroom poisoning in infants and children: the Amanita pantherina/muscaria group. J Toxicol Clin Toxicol 1992;30:12–22.

[47] Plumlee KH. Plant hazards. Vet Clin North Am Small Anim Pract 2002;32(2):383–95.

[48] Pschner B. Grayanotoxins. In: Plumlee KH, editor. Clinical veterinary toxicology. St. Louis (MO): Mosby; 2004.

[49] Castell S. Taxine alkaloids. In: Plumlee KH, editor. Clinical veterinary toxicology. St. Louis (MO): Mosby; 2004.

[50] Hall J. Lily. In: Plumlee KH, editor. Clinical veterinary toxicology. St. Louis (MO): Mosby; 2004.

[51] Fitzgerald KT. Cyanide. In: Peterson ME, Talcott PA, editors. Small animal toxicology. Philadelphia: WB Saunders; 2001.

[52] Pickerell JA, Oehme F, Mannala SA, et al. In: Plumlee KH, editor. Clinical veterinary toxicology. St. Louis (MO): Mosby; 2004.

[53] Albrectson JC. Evaluation of castor bean toxicosis in dogs. 98 cases. J Am Anim Hosp Assoc 2000;36:229–33.

[54] Albrectson JC. Cycasin. In: Plumlee KH, editor. Clinical veterinary toxicology. St. Louis (MO): Mosby; 2004.

[55] Kunkel DB, Brailberg G. Poisonous plants. In: Haddad LM, Shannon MW, Winchester JF, editors. Clinical management of poisoning and drug overdose. Philadelphia: WB Saunders; 1998.

[56] Galey D. Cardiac glycosides. In: Plumlee KH, editor. Clinical veterinary toxicology. St. Louis (MO): Mosby; 2004.

[57] Plumlee KH. Nicotine. In: Peterson ME, Talcott PA, editors. Small animal toxicology. Philadelphia: WB Saunders; 2001.

[58] Haddad LM. Nicotine. In: Haddad LM, Shannon MW, Winchester JF, editors. Clinical management of poisoning and drug overdose. Philadelphia: WB Saunders; 1998.

[59] Plumlee KH. Tannic acid. In: Plumlee KH, editor. Clinical veterinary toxicology. St. Louis (MO): Mosby; 2004.

[60] Rotstein DS, et al. Suspected oak Quercus, toxicity in an African spurred tortoise, geochelone sulcata. J Herpetol Med Surg 2003;13(3):20–1.

[61] Martin B, Szara S. Marijuana. In: Haddad LM, Shannon MW, Winchester JF, editors. Clinical management of poisoning and drug overdose. Philadelphia: WB Saunders; 1998.

[62] Volmer PA. Drugs of abuse. In: Peterson ME, Talcott PA, editors. Small animal toxicology. Philadelphia: WB Saunders; 2001.

[63] Fowler ME. Veterinary zootoxicology. Boca Raton (FL): CRC Press; 1993.

[64] Peterson ME, Talcott PA. Small animal toxicology. Philadelphia: WB Saunders; 2001.

[65] Walter FG, Fernandez MC, Haddad LM. North American venomous snakebites. In: Haddad LM, Shannon MW, Winchester JF, editors. Clinical management of poisoning and drug overdose. Philadelphia: WB Saunders; 1998.

[66] Ovadia M, Kochva E. Neutralization of Viperidae and Elapidae snake venoms by sera of different animals. Toxicon 1977;15(6):541.

[67] Philpot VB, Smith RG. Neutralization of pit viper venom by king snake serum. Proc Soc Exp Biol Med 1950;74:521.

[68] Peterson ME. Poisonous lizards. In: Peterson ME, Talcott PA, editors. Small animal toxicology. Philadelphia: WB Saunders; 2001.

[69] Fowler ME. Venomous lizards. In: Veterinary zootoxicology. Boca Raton (FL): CRC Press; 1993.

[70] Heradon RA, Tu T. Biochemical characterization of the lizard toxin gilatoxin. Biochemistry 1981;20:3517–22.

[71] Mocha-Morales J, Martin BM, Possani LD. Isolation and characterization of helothermine, a novel toxin from Helderma horridum horridum (Mexican bearded lizard) venom. Toxicon 1990;28:299–309.

[72] Peterson ME. Toad venom toxicity. In: Tilley LP, Smith WK, editors. The five-minute veterinary consult. Philadelphia: Williams & Wilkins; 1997.

[73] Peterson ME. Amphibian toxins. In: Peterson ME, Talcott PA, editors. Small animal toxicology. Philadelphia: WB Saunders; 2001.

[74] Butler VP, et al. Heterogeneity and liability of endogenous digitalis-like substances in the plasma of the toad Bufo marinus. Am J Physiol 1996;271:R325–32.

[75] Tunney FX. Stinging insects. In: Haddad LM, Shannon MW, Winchester JF, editors. Clinical management of poisoning and drug overdose. Philadelphia: WB Saunders; 1998.

[76] Tracy J, et al. The natural history of exposure to the imported fire ant (Solenopsis invicta). J Allergy Clin Immunol 1995;95:824.

[77] Eisner T, et al. Lucibufagins: defensive steroids from the fireflies. Photinus ignitus and Photinus marginellus (Coleoptera: Lampyridae). Proc Natl Acad Sci U S A 1978;75:905–8.

[78] Fieser LF, Fieser M. National products related to phenanthrene. Rheinhold (NY): Rheinhold; 1999.

[79] Glor R, et al. Two cases of firefly toxicosis in bearded dragons, Pegona vitticeps. Proc Assoc Rept Amph Vet 1999;27–30.

[80] Eisner T, et al. Firefly "femme fatales" acquire defensive steroids (lucibufagins) from their firefly prey. Proc Natl Acad Sci U S A 1997;94:9723–8.

[81] Sexton OJ. Differential predation by the lizard Anolis carolinensis on unicoloured and polycoloured insects after an interval of no contact. Anim Behav 1964;12:101–10.

[82] Lloyd JE. Firefly parasites and predators. Coleopt Bull 1998;27:91–106.

[83] Sydow SL, Lloyd JE. Distasteful fireflies sometimes emetic, but not lethal. Entomol 1998;58: 312.

[84] Case MT, et al. Acute mouse and chronic dog toxicity studies of danthron, dioctyl sodium sulfosuccinate, poloxalkol and combinations. Drug Chem Toxicol 1977–1978;1(1):89–101.

[85] Donowitz M, Binder HJ. Effect of dioctyl sodium sufosuccinate on colonic fluid and electrolyte movement. Gastroenterology 1975;69:941–50.

[86] Da Fox, et al. Surfactants selectively ablate enteric neurons of the rat jejunum. J Pharmacol Exp Ther 1983;277(2):539–44.

[87] Karlin DA, et al. Effect on dioctyl sodium sulfosuccinate feeding on rat colorectal 1, 2-dimenthylhydrazine carcinogenesis. J Natl Cancer Inst 1980;64:791–3.

[88] Lish PM. Some pharmacological effects of dioctyl sodium sulfosuccinate on the gastrointestinal tract of the rat. Toxicol Appl Pharmacol 1961;41(6):580–4.

[89] Moffatt RE, et al. Studies on dioctyl sodium sulfosuccinate toxicity: clinical, gross and microscopic pathology in the horse and guinea pig. Can J Comp Med 1975;39:434–41.

[90] Saunders DR, et al. Effect of dioctyl sodium succinate on structure and function of human and rodent intestine. Gastroenterology 1975;69(2):380–6.

[91] Paul-Murphy J, et al. Necrosis of esophageal and gastric mucosa in snakes given oral dioctyl sodium succinate. Proceedings of the 1st International Conference of Zoological and Avian Medicine, Honolulu, Hawaii; 1987.

[92] Kirk RW. Current veterinary therapy in small animal practice. Philadelphia: WB Saunders; 1976.

[93] Frye FL. Biomedical and surgical aspects of captive reptile husbandry. Edwardsville (KY): Veterinary Medical Publishing; 1981.

ELSEVIER
SAUNDERS

VETERINARY
CLINICS
Exotic Animal Practice

Vet Clin Exot Anim 11 (2008) 359–374

Toxicology of Aquarium Fish

Helen Roberts, DVM[a],*, Brian S. Palmeiro, VMD[b]

[a]*Aquatic Veterinary Services of WNY, PC, 5 Corners Animal Hospital, PC, 2799 Southwestern Blvd, Suite 100, Orchard Park, NY 14217, USA*
[b]*PetFishDoctor.com, 645 Pennsylvania Ave, Prospect Park, PA 19076, USA*

Fish have a very intimate relationship with their surrounding aquatic environment, surrendering them vulnerable to waterborne toxicities. Most aquarium fish live in a closed system (water has to be manually removed and added to be renewed), so the effects of such toxins can be cumulative and devastating. Most cases of toxicity are due to deficiencies in husbandry and tank maintenance. Poor water quality kills more fish than infectious agents, making client education a very important preventive tool for aquatic practitioners. This article includes a discussion of toxicities related to water quality, chemotherapeutics, pesticides, and household substances.

Water quality–related toxicities

Toxicities in pet fish are most commonly due to abnormalities in water quality; poor water quality is one of the most common causes of morbidity and mortality in pet fish. Therefore, a complete water quality evaluation should be performed in every case presenting to the fish veterinarian. Acute exposure to poor water quality can result in sudden and significant mortality. Chronic exposure to suboptimal water quality conditions can cause immunosuppression and predispose fish to a variety of infectious diseases that ultimately lead to mortality. Common water quality–related toxicities in aquarium fish include pH, ammonia, nitrite, nitrate, chlorine/chloramines and hydrogen sulfide.

pH toxicity

pH is the measure of hydrogen ion concentration in water. It is measured on a logarithmic scale: a change in 1 pH unit represents a tenfold difference

---

* Corresponding author.
E-mail address: nyfishdoc@aol.com (H. Roberts).

in concentration of hydrogen ions [1,2]. The pH can range from 1 to 14; values less than 7.0 are considered acidic, values greater than 7.0 are basic (alkaline), and a value of 7 is neutral. Optimal water pH varies with species. Most aquarium fish live in water with a pH ranging from 5.5 to 8.5. Fish in freshwater aquariums generally do best with a neutral pH, whereas marine fish typically require higher pH values (8.0–8.5). Some freshwater tropical fish such as discus (*Symphysodon discus*) prefer acidic water, whereas African cichlids prefer more alkaline water. A pH outside of the optimal range may not immediately result in acute mortality; however, chronic exposure may lead to stress and subsequent immunosuppression, predisposing the fish to disease.

Rapid fluctuations in pH are generally more problematic for fish than specific individual pH values. Water with low alkalinity (buffering capacity) is more likely to undergo pH fluctuations. Slow pH changes (no more than 0.3–0.5 units/d) are usually tolerated well by most fish [1]. The pH can increase during algal blooms and in heavily planted ponds/aquaria due to carbon dioxide usage [1–3]. A buildup of organic debris/organic acids can also decrease the pH of an aquarium.

Suboptimal pH or pH fluctuations can result in lethargy, stress, skin irritation/lesions, behavioral changes (such as attempting to jump out of the aquarium, flashing), corneal edema, skin color changes, gill irritation with increased mucus production, respiratory signs, and mortality [1–3]. pH swings can result in decreased immune system function, predisposing the fish to various infections (parasitic, bacterial, viral). Blood acidosis can result from decreases in pH, whereas increases in pH can result in blood alkalosis [2,3].

Regular maintenance of aquaria, including routine water changes and regular cleaning of gravel beds, is essential. In closed systems such as home aquaria, water pH gradually decreases over time due to the metabolic processes that take place.

"Old tank syndrome" is a common clinical finding that occurs in mature systems that have infrequent water changes and, often, overall neglect. A common historical finding is fish deaths after a water change. The client may also report intermittent fish deaths for no apparent reason. The tank may appear dirty or cloudy. Water chemistry testing reveals low or no alkalinity (buffering capacity), a low pH (often <5), elevated hardness, and high levels of nitrogenous waste products [1–3]. A pH crash is a term used to describe an acute decrease in water pH, and is often preceded by a drop in alkalinity. pH crashes may result in high fish mortalities (Fig. 1).

Treatment of pH abnormalities involves increasing or decreasing the pH (depending on the pH value and species involved) and improving the buffering capacity of the system. Water changes can be performed to normalize pH (the pH of the source water must be taken into consideration). Many commercial preparations/buffering compounds are available for adjusting pH. Sodium bicarbonate (baking soda) can be added at a rate of 3 mg/L

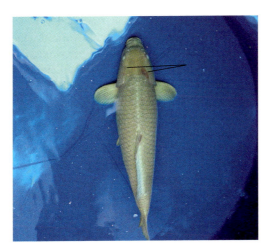

Fig. 1. A Chagoi koi (*Cyprinus carpio*) with traumatic injuries due to a pH crash. The water pH was 6.0. The black lines show area of injuries.

to temporarily improve buffering capacity/alkalinity of the system [1,2]. Long-term management of low alkalinity can be helped by the use of crushed coral, crushed oyster shells, or limestone [3]. Old tank syndrome treatments also include the use of ammonia binders, treatment of any secondary health problems, and client education in husbandry practices.

More ammonia is present in the toxic form at higher pH levels, resulting in increased ammonia toxicity. Increased toxicity of heavy metals and some medications (choramine-T, copper sulfate, formalin, malachite green) may be seen at lower pH levels [2].

Ammonia toxicity

Ammonia is the primary nitrogenous waste product of fish and also originates from the decay of complex nitrogenous/protein compounds [1,2]. Non-ionized ammonia is excreted from the gills by diffusion. Environmental increases in non-ionized ammonia decrease the rate of diffusion from the gills, resulting in elevated blood and tissue ammonia levels. Ammonia toxicity is one of the most common water quality problems affecting aquarium fish and can cause acute mortality or chronic sublethal stress. Nitrifying bacteria oxidize ammonia to nitrites and nitrites to nitrates. New tanks or ponds that lack nitrifying bacteria (an "immature" biofilter) have an increase in nitrogenous compounds ("new tank syndrome") that resolves as the biofilter matures.

Ammonia is present in two forms: ionized (NH_4^+) and non-ionized (also called un-ionized, NH_3). Non-ionized ammonia is the most toxic form. The portion of total environmental ammonia that is present in the non-ionized form is dependent on pH and, to a lesser degree, on water temperature and salinity. Ammonia is more toxic in warmer water, at higher pH, and at lower salinity [1–3]. The higher the pH, the more ammonia is present in the non-ionized form; therefore, ammonia toxicity is worsened in aquaria that have higher pH. For every 1-unit decrease in pH, there is a tenfold decrease in non-ionized ammonia [2].

Ammonia toxicity can result from overcrowding, overfeeding, buildup of organic debris, infrequent water changes, immature/inadequate biologic filtration as seen in new tank syndrome, or damage to existing biofiltration (vigorous cleaning, certain medications). Clinical signs of ammonia toxicity include mortalities, neurologic and behavioral abnormalities, lethargy, anorexia, poor growth, secondary infections, injected fins, and respiratory signs due to gill hyperplasia/hypertrophy [1–3]. The precise mechanism of ammonia poisoning in fish is unknown; however, high aqueous ammonia increases blood and tissue ammonia levels, causing elevated blood pH, osmoregulatory disturbance, increased tissue oxygen consumption, and decreased blood oxygen transport [2]. Ammonia toxicity causes branchial irritation resulting in gill hyperplasia, hypertrophy, and hypoxia [2,4]. Neurologic signs can develop, likely due to interference with neurotransmitters in the brain [4].

Diagnosis of ammonia toxicity is easily attained using commercially available test kits (Fig. 2); these kits typically report total ammonia nitrogen. The concentration of non-ionized ammonia can be determined from a standard chart depending on temperature and pH. Any value of ammonia should be regarded as significant. Ammonia tolerance varies with species but it is generally recommended that ammonia levels measure 0 mg/L to maintain healthy aquarium fish.

Frequent water changes (30%–50%) are the mainstay of treatment of ammonia toxicity. Feeding should be decreased or temporarily stopped. In overcrowded aquariums, the stocking density should be decreased. The pH should be evaluated and maintained; an increase toward the alkaline range of normal pH should be avoided. Good oxygenation should be

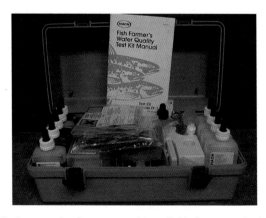

Fig. 2. An example of a water test kit available from www.hach.com.

maintained. Commercial ammonia binders are available but may interfere with ammonia test kits that use Nessler reagent. In any case of ammonia toxicity, the life-support system (or systems) should be evaluated and improved if necessary [5]. If chemical treatment results in biofilter damage, then activated carbon can be used to remove the drug from the system. Low doses of salt increase the ionization of ammonia and decrease toxicity [1,2,5].

Nitrite toxicity (brown blood disease, methemoglobinemia)

Ammonia is oxidized to nitrite (NO_2^-) by *Nitrosomonas* and other microbes. Causes for elevated nitrite in aquaria are similar to those listed under ammonia toxicity, and elevated nitrite is common in new tank syndrome (with a maturing biofilter). Clinical signs of nitrite toxicity in fish are predominantly respiratory in nature and include increased opercular rate, piping (gasping at surface), gathering in well-aerated areas (eg, near filter input), and death [1–3]. Nitrite is absorbed by the gills and oxidizes hemoglobin to methemoglobin, resulting in methemoglobinemia and hypoxia. Gills may appear pale or tan in color. In severe cases, gills and blood may show brown discoloration due to the methemoglobin [1–3].

Nitrite toxicity is best diagnosed by finding elevated nitrite in the aquarium combined with elevated methemoglobin levels in the blood [6]. More commonly it is diagnosed with compatible clinical signs and elevated nitrite levels on commercial test kits. The optimal level of nitrite in aquarium water is 0 mg/L.

Treatment of nitrite toxicity is similar to treatment of ammonia toxicity (water changes, feeding and stocking density decreases, biofiltration improvement, and so forth). Oxygenation should be improved to improve the relative degree of hypoxia. Most freshwater fishes actively transport nitrite from the water by way of the chloride uptake mechanism on chloride cells of the gills. The rate of uptake can vary depending on the water temperature, pH, and chloride level. Toxicity can be prevented or treated by adding chloride (as sodium chloride) to the water [6]. Due to higher levels of chloride in seawater, marine fish are less sensitive to nitrite toxicity [2].

Nitrate toxicity

Nitrite is oxidized to nitrate (NO_3) by *Nitrobacter* and other microbes. It is the least toxic of the nitrogenous compounds, but eggs and fry may be more sensitive to toxicity than adult fish. The most common cause for elevated nitrates is infrequent water changes; other causes are similar to those listed for ammonia toxicity. Clinical signs of nitrate toxicity include poor growth, lethargy, anorexia, opportunistic infections, and injected fins [1–3]. One study suggested that prolonged exposure to elevated nitrate levels

ROBERTS & PALMEIRO

might result in a pathologic response demonstrated by biochemical and hematologic changes [7]. Although the investigators could not conclusively prove that high nitrate levels were responsible for the changes, the results were highly suggestive [7]. High levels of nitrate can encourage algal blooms that can result in other water quality abnormalities (Fig. 3). The diagnosis can be confirmed with commercial test kits; nitrate levels should be maintained below 50 mg/L. Treatment for nitrate toxicity involves frequent water changes and removing organic debris. Aquatic plants can remove some nitrates from the water but do not eliminate the need for water changes and routine cleaning [1,3].

Chlorine and chloramine toxicity

Chlorine is added to municipal water to kill microorganisms and is highly toxic to fish [2]. The average level of chlorine in municipal tap water can vary between 0.5 ppm and 2.0 ppm. Chloramines (formed by a reaction between ammonia and chlorine) may also be used as disinfectants in municipal water supplies and are toxic to fish [2]. Chorine causes gill necrosis resulting in hypoxia [2]. Chlorine and chloramine can also result in hemolytic anemia [4]. Chloramine may result in methemoglobin formation by oxidizing hemoglobin to methemoglobin [4]. The most common cause of chlorine/chloramine toxicity in aquarium fish occurs when water is added without prior dechlorination. Fish affected by chlorine toxicity typically exhibit respiratory signs and acute mortality [1,2]. Chronic exposure to lower levels of chlorine may result in a history of sporadic mortalities. Sunken eyes have been reported as a possible clinical sign in cases of chronic exposure [6].

Commercial test kits for chlorine and chloramines are available and aid in the diagnosis of chlorine/chloramine toxicity. Chlorine is easily removed from water with dechlorinators such as sodium thiosulfate (3.5 mg/L) or by aeration of water for 24 hours in an open-topped container [1,2].

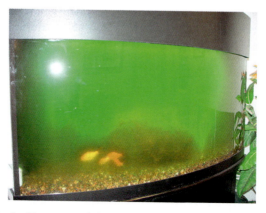

Fig. 3. Algae accumulation in a tank due to high nitrate levels.

Dechlorinators (like sodium thiosulfate) remove the chlorine from chloramines and release ammonia into the water [2]. The resulting ammonia is usually handled by the biofiltration in life-support systems unless the biofilter is immature, such as in a new aquarium setup. Fish treated for acute chlorine toxicity have improved survival if the water is supersaturated with oxygen; lowering the water temperature may also be beneficial [2].

Hydrogen sulfide toxicity

Hydrogen sulfide (H_2S) is produced from the reduction of sulfate ion under anaerobic conditions [2]. It can occur at the bottom of aquaria that have excessive organic debris or in deep gravel or sand filter beds that are not completely aerated (Fig. 4). Hydrogen sulfide toxicity is more of an issue in brackish and marine systems due to increased concentration of sulfate ions [2]. Disturbing the filter media or bottom substrate, which can occur when an owner vigorously cleans the gravel bed after a long period of neglecting routine maintenance, can release hydrogen sulfide into the water column. The owner may report a "black cloud" released into the water during this cleaning. Hydrogen sulfide may also be present in well water. Hydrogen sulfide interferes with respiratory function and results in hypoxia [1–3]. Affected fish demonstrate lethargy, anorexia, respiratory signs, and sudden death [1–3].

Presence of hydrogen sulfide can be detected by its characteristic rotten egg odor and can be confirmed with commercial test kits. Any levels detectable with commercial test kits should be considered detrimental [2]. Aggressive aeration and water changes remove hydrogen sulfide from the water. Maintaining aerobic environments in the tank and filter by removing decomposing detritus and allowing for thorough aeration of the filter bed prevents hydrogen sulfide accumulation. A degassing tower can be used to remove hydrogen sulfide from the water before it comes into contact with the fish. Potassium permanganate (2 mg/L) oxides/detoxifies hydrogen

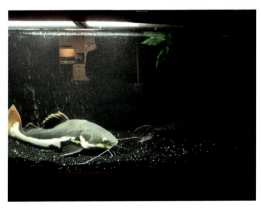

Fig. 4. A deep layer of gravel in a 180-gal tank. Unless maintained, the gravel bed can develop pockets of hydrogen sulfide gas.

sulfide but cannot be used in marine systems [2]. Increasing the pH and lowering the temperature also decreases hydrogen sulfide toxicity [2]. Caution should be taken when restarting filters that have been turned off, because anaerobic environments may have been created.

Chemotherapeutic toxicities

Improperly administered chemical treatments can be a cause of toxicity in aquarium fish. In many cases, treatment dosages are based on empiric and anecdotal information; toxicity may therefore occur at recommended dosages. Pharmacokinetic data are seldom available for agents used to treat ornamental fish. Susceptibility to chemotherapeutic toxicity varies with species, water quality, and medication used. Chemotherapeutics can damage the biofilter, the fish, and other organisms that inhabit the aquarium. Common chemotherapeutics that can result in toxicity in aquarium fish include copper, formalin, potassium permanganate, malachite green, quaternary ammonium compounds, organophosphates, and antibiotics such as gentamicin, sulfonamides, and oxytetracycline.

Copper toxicity

Copper (most commonly as copper sulfate) is used in the treatment of various ectoparasites in aquarium fish. It has a narrow therapeutic index, and accurate dosing is critical to prevent toxicity. Free copper ions must be maintained between 0.15 mg/L and 0.20 mg/L [2]. Copper is primarily toxic to the gill tissue, resulting in osmoregulatory dysfunction and hypoxia [2,3]. It may also damage the kidney and liver and result in immunosuppression [2]. Copper is extremely toxic to invertebrates. Copper toxicity can also result from the use of copper piping or decorations. Toxicity is most common in systems with low alkalinity, especially with low pH [5]. Copper treatments are not recommended in systems with a total alkalinity of less than 50 mg/L; in general, the authors do not recommend copper treatment in freshwater systems, especially when safer alternatives exist.

Clinical signs of copper toxicity include lethargy, anorexia, and respiratory signs [2,3] in addition to abnormal behavior, gill edema, disorientation, and scale protrusion [6]. Some species of fish may also show intense coloration before death [6]. Diagnosis of copper toxicity is made by way of history and commercial test kits. When copper toxicity occurs, large water changes and oxygenation of the water should be performed. Copper toxicity can be prevented by carefully monitoring copper levels and by avoiding its use in systems that have low alkalinity.

Formalin toxicity

Formalin is an aqueous solution of 37% formaldehyde gas [2,3]. It is used to treat a variety of ectoparasites in ornamental fish, most commonly at the concentration of 25 mg/L (1 mL/10 gal). Formalin decreases dissolved oxygen in the water and can cause irritation of the gills; therefore, water should be oxygenated well during treatment. Formalin is more toxic in soft, acidic water and at higher temperatures [2]. A recent study evaluating the tolerance of various disinfectants in common aquarium fish found that goldfish (*Carassius auratus*) are more sensitive to the effects of formalin than zebrafish (*Danio rerio*) [8]. Exposure to formalin at a reported therapeutic dosage (250 ppm for 1 hour) resulted in toxic effects in goldfish but not in zebrafish, and prolonged exposure increased toxicity in goldfish but not in zebrafish [8]. The median lethal dose (LD_{50}) was 648 ppm for 1 hour in zebrafish and 272 ppm for 1 hour in goldfish [8].

Fish affected by formalin toxicity typically illustrate respiratory signs (eg, piping), decreased activity, loss of equilibrium, erratic swimming, excess mucus production, color changes, and mortality [2,3,8]. Treatment of formalin toxicity involves water changes, removing excess formalin with activated carbon, and aggressive aeration of the water. Formalin should never be used when the preparation appears cloudy or has a white precipitate. Formalin is a carcinogen and should be handled carefully [2].

Potassium permanganate

Potassium permanganate (K-P) is an oxidizing agent used to treat a variety of ectoparasites and external skin/gill bacterial infections in freshwater fish [2]. Effective treatment concentration requires 2 mg/L of active chemical; permanganate ion imparts a light pink or purple color to the water that fades as it becomes inactive [2]. Exposure of goldfish and zebrafish to lethal concentrations of potassium permanganate resulted in decreased activity, loss of equilibrium, erratic swimming, and death [8]. Goldfish were less sensitive to the effects of potassium permanganate then zebrafish; the LD_{50} was 5.75 ppm for 1 hour in zebrafish and greater than 25 ppm for 1 hour in goldfish [8]. Prolonged exposure increased toxicity in zebrafish but not in goldfish [8]. Potassium permanganate is toxic in water that has high pH because manganese dioxide may precipitate onto the gills; therefore, it should not be used in marine systems [2]. Potassium permanganate is extremely toxic when mixed with formalin [2].

Malachite green

Malachite green is a diarylmethane dye that is effective in the treatment of water mold infections and some ectoparasites in fish [2]. It is also a respiratory poison, teratogen, and suspected carcinogen and should be handled with caution [2]. Toxicity in fish typically presents as respiratory distress, given its activity as a metabolic respiratory poison [2]. Malachite green is reported as being hepatotoxic and implicated in causing developmental abnormalities when used to treat fish eggs [3]. Signs of malachite green toxicity in zebrafish and goldfish include decreased activity, loss of equilibrium, erratic swimming, and death [8]. Extending the treatment time enhanced toxicity in goldfish but not in zebrafish [8]. The LD_{50} was 8.68 ppm for 30 minutes in zebrafish and 9.23 ppm for 30 minutes in goldfish [8]. The toxicity of malachite green increases with higher temperatures and with lower pH [2]. Some species such as tetras, catfish, and loaches are reportedly more sensitive to malachite green toxicity [2]. Young fry and near-hatching eggs are also very sensitive to toxicity [2]. Malachite green can be removed from the system with water changes and activated carbon.

Quaternary ammonium compounds

Quaternary ammonium compounds, such as benzalkonium chlorides and benzethonium chlorides, are disinfectants that may be used as antiseptics to treat external infections in fish [2]. Quaternary ammonium compounds are more toxic at higher temperatures and in softer water [2]. In one study, benzalkonium chloride was tolerated well by goldfish and by zebrafish [8]. There was no mortality in any of the fish exposed to benzalakonium chloride at or below the therapeutic dosage (2.0 ppm for 1 hour) [8]. Signs of toxicity occurred with greater than three times the therapeutic concentration and included decreased activity and loss of equilibrium [8]. The LD_{50} was 6.28 ppm for 1 hour in zebrafish and 5.80 ppm for 1 hour in goldfish [8].

Organophosphate toxicity

Organophosphates have been widely used for the treatment of ectoparasites in aquarium fish. These compounds are also potentially harmful to humans. In most cases, safer alternative treatments are available. Many species are sensitive to the toxic effects of organophosphates, even when therapeutic doses are used. Until the 1970s, dichlorvos (or dichlorvos mixtures) was used to control common carp populations by fisheries biologists [9]. The toxic effects of organophosphates in fish manifest primarily as neurologic signs. Clinical signs of organophosphate toxicity include vertebral fractures, convulsions, respiratory difficulty, erratic swimming movements, weakness or restlessness, and mortalities [2,10]. Because the use of trichlorphon, fenthion, and dichlorvos is extensively described in the literature and in hobbyist texts, the aquatic practitioner may still see toxicities from these agents. There is no specific treatment for organophosphate toxicity. Surviving exposed fish should be moved to clean water.

Antibiotics

Aquatic practitioners frequently use antibiotics to treat a variety of infectious maladies. In addition, antibiotics are readily available to hobbyists over-the-counter, potentially leading to inappropriate dosing and toxicity.

Pharmacokinetic data are not available for many drugs, and effective therapeutic dosing regimens can vary widely among fish species. Anecdotal data and extrapolation from the drugs used in other species may be used to treat fish patients. The potential for adverse side effects may also be extrapolated from use in other species. The common use of parenteral antibiotics and the frequent alterations in dosing regimens (usually shorter intervals and higher dosages) among laymen can increase the potential for toxic side effects. Questioning the owner on the use of previous therapeutants is an essential part of the historical data gathered on a sick fish consult. Aminoglycosides such as kanamycin, amikacin, and gentamicin have been documented to be nephrotoxic in several species. Nephrotoxicity may even occur at therapeutic doses, depending on the species [2,3]. Oxytetracycline can be immunotoxic in several species [2,11], and degraded products may be nephrotoxic [2]. In addition, the use of antibiotics as a prolonged immersion treatment may adversely affect biofiltration, leading to water quality concerns.

Pesticide toxicities

Aquarium fish are less likely to encounter pesticide toxicities than their farmed and wild cousins, but toxicities can still occur. Most household pesticides are highly toxic to fish. Organophosphates, chlorinated hydrocarbons, pyrethrins, and pyrethroids make up the most likely suspects in pesticide toxicity cases. Indoor pest extermination most likely involves aerosol spraying procedures, so it is important for the homeowner to turn off air pumps and cover the tank until the danger of pesticide introduction has passed. Although rare, curious household pets have been known to fall into tanks and indoor ponds. If these pets have had a recent application of a topical pesticide or are wearing an insecticide-impregnated collar, toxicity in the tank may occur. Clinical signs vary but are mostly neurologic in nature. Acute reactions include paralysis and death [3]. Chronic exposure has been associated with poor growth and deformities in fry [3]. Vertebral fractures have also been reported [2].

Household toxicities

In general, few household toxicities present with pathognomonic lesions. Some identification of the toxin may be gained by carefully questioning the owner. In situations in which accidental contamination of the aquaria is suspected, the goals of treatment are to move the fish to clean, uncontaminated water and to provide symptomatic therapy such as additional aeration, treatment of secondary infections, and reduction of stress. In cases in which the fish cannot be removed, frequent, ample water changes should be recommended. Water quality should also be monitored in case of filter failure. Education of the owner may help to mitigate potentially disastrous situations. Many owners are unfamiliar with proper breakdown, disinfection, and cleaning procedures of used tanks and equipment (nets, decoration, siphon pumps, and so forth). Listed below are some common scenarios that may occur in home aquaria.

Nicotine

Cigarette smoke fumes containing several toxins, including nicotine, can be introduced into a fish tank by an air pump, whereby they are rapidly absorbed into the water. Nicotine is soluble in water and very toxic to fish [2,3,6]. Guppies exposed to a smoky room for 1 hour experienced high mortalities [6]. Clinical signs of nicotine toxicity include abnormal posture (rigid pectoral fins, clamped fins), muscular spasms, pale coloration, and death [6]. Chronic exposure to low doses can cause deformed fry and infertility [6]. Treatment is general and aimed at removing the fish from the toxic environment. Frequent water changes, fresh activated carbon, or placing the fish in a fresh tank may reduce the impact of nicotine.

Detergents

Most cleaning agents and detergents used in homes are extremely toxic to fish [3]. Several household cleaners contain detergents and several other compounds, including ammonia-based products. Detergents may find entry into home aquaria by way of aerosol dispersion, accidental spillage, and intentional use by the owner. Failure to thoroughly rinse aquaria equipment and tanks is a common problem that can lead to toxicity in fish. Cationic detergents may contain quaternary ammonium disinfectants, another group of toxic compounds to fish [6]. Detergents break down the protective mucus layer on fish skin, facilitating pathogen entry [6]. Clinical signs of detergent contamination include skin hemorrhages, flashing due to irritation, excess mucus production or "dry skin" due to epithelial disruption, and edema of the gill epithelium [2]. Foam and bubbles may still be visible on the water surface. Treatment involves moving fish to fresh, oxygenated water. Salt at 0.1% may be added to freshwater to reduce stress.

Food-related toxicities

Food-related toxicities occur due to spoilage of food, contamination of food, the addition of potentially toxic ingredients to food, improperly balanced diets, and an inadvertent excess (toxic) amount of a required nutrient. In light of the recent pet food recall scares of 2005 (aflatoxin-contaminated dry pet food) and 2007 (melamine and cyanuric acid toxic reaction), consumers are more conscious of what is being fed to their pets, including their pet fish. One only has to visit the pet store, read trade journals, or look online to see the huge variety of foods available for feeding pet fish. Pet fish food is available frozen, live, pelleted, flaked, baked, and soft-moist, among other preparations. Despite the scrutiny, food-related toxicities still occasionally occur.

Aflatoxins are mycotoxins produced by *Aspergillus* spp, molds that occur commonly in the environment. Foods that are most susceptible to aflatoxin contamination are those containing oilseed crops (corn, cottonseed, and peanut meal), but other grains and feed are also susceptible [12]. The feed is more likely to have increased amounts of aflatoxin when stored at high temperature and humidity levels and when it has a high moisture content. Aflatoxin causes hepatotoxicity, and with prolonged feeding at sublethal levels, it can lead to hepatic neoplasia [2,4,12–14]. Sensitivity varies with species. Clinical signs of aflatoxicosis range from decreased growth or lack of weight gain, pale gills/anemia, and impaired coagulation (Fig. 5) [12]. Aflatoxin can also destroy important nutrients in food, such as thiamine and vitamins A and C [12]. Subsequent immunosuppression can lead to increased susceptibility to other diseases [12]. As part of an environmental assessment and complete history, the owner should be questioned on feeding habits for the pet fish. When there is a high index of suspicion for aflatoxicosis, a sample of food can be evaluated by a diagnostic laboratory. It is wise to contact the laboratory before sending any samples to verify whether the test can be performed and to determine the specifics of sample submission.

In 2007, a nationwide recall of dog and cat food occurred because of the addition of melamine and cyanuric acid. When both ingredients were present in the food, crystals formed that potentially impaired renal function, sometimes leading to renal failure and death [15]. One large pet product company also voluntarily recalled several varieties of fish food due to potential melamine contamination [16]. No fish toxicities were reported due to the use of commercial diets during this recall.

Some plant legume proteins that contain nonessential amino acids have been found to be toxic when fed to fish, resulting in reduced growth [13]. The essential amino acid leucine has been reported to cause toxicity in

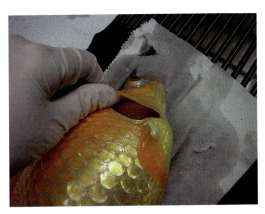

Fig. 5. Examination of pale gills in a goldfish (*Carassius auratus*).

rainbow trout. Clinical signs include scoliosis, deformed scales and opercula, and epidermal spongiosis [13]. The fat-soluble vitamins A, D, and E can cause toxicity when consumed in excess by fish. Salmonids were reported to experience decreased growth and reduced red cell counts [13]. In addition, toxic consumption of vitamin A resulted in necrosis of fins and tail, scoliosis, lordosis, pale yellow livers, and increased mortalities in salmonids [13].

Ingredients used to manufacture food may be contaminated with residues of pesticides, herbicides, and heavy metals [13]. Contamination by various toxins may also occur. These toxins are derived from protozoans, algae, fungi, and bacteria [13]. Pathogenic bacteria, parasites, and viruses are a risk when feeding live foods.

Heavy metal toxicities

Heavy metals that cause toxicity in aquarium fish include copper, zinc, mercury, cadmium, lead, and aluminum. Heavy metals usually originate in the water supply [3]. Older plumbing can leach metals into the water source of aquaria, especially after pipes have not been used for a period of time, allowing a higher concentration of metal to develop. Other sources include inappropriate tank décor, therapeutic agents (copper) [3], runoff, and contamination of ground water in wells. The level of toxicity depends on the water pH, hardness, temperature, and the presence of organic material and solids [2,3,6]. In general, heavy metals are more toxic at lower pH, at higher temperatures, in soft water, and at low alkalinity levels. Zinc toxicity may present in koi (*Cyprinus carpio*) that are wintered-over in galvanized tubs or live in indoor display ponds into which coins are thrown by the public. Copper and zinc toxicity effects are additive. High iron levels in water can lead to the precipitation of iron oxides. A heavy layer of iron oxides on the gills can lead to lamellar fusion and to severe gill disease [4]. Clinical signs of iron toxicity reflect the relative hypoxia (piping, gasping, and increased opercular rate). Rust-colored staining of tanks, gravel, and other aquarium equipment may be seen when performing an environmental evaluation. Lead toxicity may be caused by the use of lead plant weights, lead plumbing, lead paint, and lead solder joints [2]. Clinical indications of lead toxicity in some species of fish include scoliosis, anemia and stippling of the red blood cells, lordosis, and black tail (caudal cutaneous melanosis) [2,13]. Heavy metals affect the gills, kidneys, and liver [3], and clinical signs may reflect the extent of damage to these organs in exposed fish. Respiratory difficulty and osmoregulatory disturbances are the most common signs observed.

Definitive diagnosis requires submission of a water sample to an environmental or analytic laboratory. Source water should also be evaluated. Affected fish can also be submitted to analytic laboratories in cases of suspected heavy metal poisoning [2]. Specific handling instructions are required for processing the samples to prevent contamination or an inaccurate diagnosis [2]. Treatment of heavy metal toxicity requires identifying and removing the source of exposure. No specific treatment with chelating agents or anti-dotes has been fully evaluated [6], although the use of EDTA has been recommended in the literature [2]. Water that has elevated iron levels can be pumped through an ion exchange filter before use in tanks [2].

Miscellaneous toxicities

Cyanide

Fish are very sensitive to the toxic effects of cyanide. Many species of common marine aquarium fish are collected outside the United States with the use of cyanide. Cyanide fishing has been reported to cause reef loss and deaths in smaller, nontarget fish [17]. Cyanide toxicity can also result from the use of salt containing yellow prussiate of soda (sodium ferrocyanide), an anticaking ingredient added to water conditioner. Clinical signs of acute toxicity include impaired swimming ability and relative performance, susceptibility to predation, muscle tremors, disrupted respiration, osmoregulatory disturbances, and altered growth patterns [18]. Clinical signs of hypoxia and stress can also be seen. The toxic effects from cyanide fishing may be further enhanced by hypoxic periods experienced during the transportation and handling of fish from the site of collection to wholesale distributors and, eventually, to the retailer [19]. Exposure to low levels of cyanide can cause poor reproductive performance and liver damage [19]. Owners may notice mortalities in cyanide-collected fish a short time after their introduction to the aquarium. Although clinical signs of toxicity may not precede the mortalities, hepatic necrosis, suggestive of cyanide exposure, can be detected on histopathologic examination.

Algicides (pseudo-poisoning)

Although not a true toxicity, the use of commercially available algicides can result in fish deaths. It is not unusual for an aquatic practitioner to receive a frantic phone call from an owner wondering whether the algicide used was toxic to the fish. Most fatalities can be attributed to acute low dissolved oxygen content following algal death. Decaying oxygen consumes a large amount of dissolved oxygen in the water [2]. If the pre-existing dissolved oxygen was borderline or low, then the resulting algal decay can wreak havoc in a system. An algae crash or widespread algae death for other reasons can also result in a similar situation.

References

[1] Palmeiro BS, Shelton J. Water quality and pet fish health. In: Mayer J, editor. Five minute veterinary consult: exotic animal medicine. Ames (IA): Blackwell Publishing; 2008, in press.
[2] Noga EJ. Fish disease: diagnosis and treatment. St. Louis (MO): Mosby; 1996.
[3] Wildgoose WH. BSAVA manual of ornamental fish. 2nd edition. Quedgeley, Gloucester (UK): British Small Animal Veterinary Association; 2001.

[4] Ferguson HW. Systemic pathology of fish. 2nd edition. London: Scotian Press; 2006.
[5] Hadfield CA, Whitaker BR, Clayton LA. Emergency and critical care of fish. Vet Clin North Am Exot Anim 2007;10:647–55.
[6] Stoskopf MK. Fish medicine. Philadelphia: WB Saunders; 1993.
[7] Hrubec TC, Smith SA, Robertson JL. Nitrate toxicity: a potential problem of recirculating systems. Successes and Failures in Commercial Recirculating Aquaculture 1996;1:41–8.
[8] Intorre L, Meucci VM, DiBello D, et al. Tolerance of benzalkonium chloride, formalin, malachite green, and potassium permanganate in goldfish and zebrafish. J Am Vet Med Assoc 2007;231(4):590–5.
[9] ASTDR. Agency for Toxic Substances and Disease Registry. Toxicologic Profile for Dichlorvos, September 1997. Section 4, Production, Import Use and Disposal. p. 126. Available at: http://www.atsdr.cdc.gov/. Accessed September 24, 2007.
[10] Murphy I, Lewbart GA, Meerdink GL, et al. Whole-blood and plasma cholinesterase levels in normal koi (Cyprinus carpio). J Vet Diagn Invest 2005;17:74–5.
[11] Boon JH, van der Heijden MHT, Tanck MWT, et al. Effects of antibacterial drugs on European eel (Anguilla anguilla L., 1758) peripheral leucocytes. Comp Haematol Int 1995; 5(4):268–72.
[12] Russo J-AR, Yanong RPE. Molds in fish feeds and aflatoxins. Institute of Food and Agricultural Sciences. University of Florida Fact Sheet FA-95; 2006. Available at: http://edis.ifas.ufl.edu. Accessed September 14, 2007.
[13] Tacon AGJ. Nutritional fish pathology. Morphological signs of nutrient deficiency and toxicity in farmed fish. FAO (Food and Agricultural Organization of the United Nations) Technical Paper No 330. Rome: FAO; 1992.
[14] Johnson D. Practical koi and goldfish medicine. Exot DVM 2004;6(3):42–8.
[15] University Of Guelph. Pet food recall: how melamine impairs kidney function. Science Daily 2007. Available at: http://www.sciencedaily.com/releases/2007/05/070501105514.htm. Accessed October 31, 2007.
[16] Atlantis fish flake food voluntary recall. In: Pet Health News-August 2007. Sergeant's Pet Care Products, Inc.; Available at: http://www.sergeants.com/atlantisinfo/index.asp. Accessed September 25, 2007.
[17] Mous PJ, Pet-Soede L, Erdmann M, et al. Cyanide fishing on Indonesian coral reefs for the live food fish market—What is the problem? Conservation and Community Investment Forum (CCIF) [Internet], San Francisco. 2000. Available at: http://www.cciforum.org/pdfs/Cyanide_fishing1.pdf. Accessed September 16, 2007.
[18] Eisler R. Cyanide hazards to fish, wildlife, and invertebrates: a synoptic review. U.S. Fish and Wildlife Service, Patuxent Wildlife Research Center, Laurel (MD). Contaminant Hazard Reviews Biological Report 1991;85(1.23).
[19] Speare DJ. Liver diseases of tropical fish. Semin Avian Exot Pet Med 2000;9(3):174–8.

ELSEVIER
SAUNDERS

Vet Clin Exot Anim 11 (2008) 375–387

VETERINARY
CLINICS
Exotic Animal Practice

Toxic Exotics

Michael E. Peterson, DVM, MS[a,b,*]

[a]Reid Veterinary Hospital, 933 SW Queen Avenue, Albany, OR 97321, USA
[b]College of Veterinary Medicine, Oregon State University, Corvallis, OR 97331-4801, USA

In today's society with Internet access to numerous wholesale and retail animal markets, many owners have obtained various dangerous exotic "pets." This "underground zoo" is more significant than the average veterinary practitioner might imagine. Anyone can sit at a computer and, within a matter of a few minutes, purchase gaboon vipers, puff adders, cobras (spitting or not), and many other venomous creatures. In many major cities, these animals can even be purchased at swap meets or herptatologic society meetings. A query of the fire and police departments of any major city can confirm the presence and size of the underground zoo. The purpose of this article is to familiarize the reader with the basic venom components, the pathophysiologic responses of envenomated dogs and cats, and some brief treatment guidelines for envenomations by various exotic "pets." The growing trend toward the collection of exotic animals by private owners increases the likelihood that veterinarians will face the challenge of treating an exotic envenomation.

The increasing popularity of venomous exotics as captive pets predicates the need for private collectors to have a pre-existing treatment strategy with their local emergency centers. Such arrangements may facilitate the treatment of envenomation by these exotic pets. One benefit is that the owners usually know exactly what species of animal has done the envenomating.

When treating an exotic envenomation, the veterinary clinician should contact personnel at the regional poison control center. They are prepared to assist by facilitating the timely acquisition of exotic antivenins by accessing the updated antivenin index. This access allows them to provide information 24 hours a day to help locate the nearest appropriate antivenin for all snakes indigenous to the United States and exotic snakes found in zoologic gardens. Any regional Poison Control Center can be reached by

* Reid Veterinary Hospital, 933 SW Queen Avenue, Albany, OR 97321.
  E-mail address: petersonkate@netscape.net

telephone at 1-800-222-1222. They also can arrange consultation with experts experienced in the management and treatment of exotic envenomations. Zoos are usually required to stock antivenins for each of their venomous exhibits. Allergic reactions to the antivenin are possible, and the clinician should be prepared to respond to severe reactions (although they are rare).

The breakdown of species to be covered in this article is general, and representative species are discussed. Included are reptiles, amphibians, and arthropods. Australian species are very toxic but difficult to import; therefore, they are not included in this review.

Reptiles

Snakes—Elapidae (fixed front fangs)

Early administration of antivenin prevents respiratory paralysis after elapid snake bite. Patients that have evidence of respiratory insufficiency after neurotoxic venom poisoning require rapid intubations and artificial ventilation. Anticholinesterase agents may help reverse neuromuscular dysfunction caused by elapid envenoming and may accelerate recovery.

Cobra

A cobra is technically any species from the genus *Naja*, but this name is commonly used to describe several snake species that spread their "hood." Examples are the king cobra (*Ophiophagus hannah*) and the ringhals (*Haemachatus*). Some African cobra species, known as the spitting cobras, have modified fangs that allow the venom to be ejected forward up to 3 m.

Envenomation from cobra bites causes major morbidity and mortality in Asia and Africa. Victims may develop cranial neuropathy, respiratory failure, and coagulopathy. Onset of clinical signs can be delayed for hours. Respiratory failure often necessitates endotracheal intubation and edrophonium and polyvalent antivenin administration. Necrosis is typical of bites by the African spitting cobras (*Naja nigricollis, Naja mossambica, Naja pallida,* and *Naja katiensis*), the Chinese cobra (*Naja atra*), the monocellate cobra (*Naja kaouthia*), and the Sumatran spitting cobra (*Naja sumatrana*). Although the venoms of these cobras contain neurotoxins, necrosis often is the chief or only manifestation of envenoming in humans. Anticholinesterases are beneficial in the management of neurotoxic envenomation by Asian cobras (*Naja naja*). Antivenins are largely ineffective in preventing the necrosis caused by many cobra venoms.

King cobra

King cobra (*Ophiophagus hannah*) envenomations induce a rapid, progressive neurotoxicity that is manifested clinically by bulbar and respiratory paralysis requiring endotracheal intubation and mechanical support. Antivenins are available.

Krait

The Malayan krait (*Bungarus candidus*) is one of the most medically significant snake species in Southeast Asia. No specific antivenin exists to treat envenomation by this species. Death can occur within 30 minutes after its bite due to the presence of highly lethal postsynaptic neurotoxins in the venom of these snakes. The venom component α-bungarotoxin appears to be widely present and conserved in Southeast and East Asian black-and-white kraits across populations and taxa.

Envenomation by the Chinese krait (*Bungarus multicinctus*) produces minimal local reactions. Onset of neurotoxic symptoms can occur several hours after the bite, and the interval between bite and death often ranges from 12 to 30 hours. Deaths are due to respiratory failure. Mildly envenomed cases may recover spontaneously without assisted ventilation. Severely envenomated patients may recover after several days of intensive respiratory care.

Victims bitten by the Malayan krait (*Bungarus candidus*) develop ptosis and generalized muscle weakness that can progress to respiratory paralysis. Evidence of decreased parasympathetic activity manifested by mydriasis, hypertension, and tachycardia may also become evident. In some human patients, hypertension resolved 6 to 60 days after admission; mydriasis and tachycardia persisted between 7 days and 2 years after discharge in all patients [1]. One patient had constipation and defects in micturition that persisted 2 years after the bite. Often, abdominal pain developed within hours of the bite. Autonomic disturbances including transient hypertension, tachycardia, lacrimation, sweating, and salivation occurred in 139 (66%) human patients who had moderate to severe envenomation [2]. Mortality can be minimized with early access to mechanical ventilation.

Mamba

The black mamba (*Dendroaspis polylepis*) is an exotic snake native to Southeast Africa with a high potential for lethality. It is estimated that two drops of venom can be fatal to an adult human. Before antivenin was available, 100% of envenomations were fatal. Clinical signs include twitching, pallor, and combativeness. Drowsiness, neurologic and neuromuscular symptoms may develop early; paralysis, ventilatory failure, or death often ensue rapidly. Victims frequently require intubations. The clinical course can include wound necrosis.

Green mamba envenomations can also induce pronounced cardiovascular problems.

Coral snake

The coral snakes are New World elapids of the genus *Micrurus*. Color pattern distinctions used for North American coral snakes (black on yellow, and so forth) do not translate to Central and South American coral snake species.

The venom is primarily neurotoxic and induces a curarelike syndrome, the onset of which can be several hours post envenomation. This syndrome begins with alterations in mental status, generalized weakness, and muscle fasciculations. Progression to paralysis follows; death is due to respiratory failure. In canine victims, marked hemolysis causing severe anemia and hemoglobinuria may develop.

There is generally good cross-reactivity with coral snake antivenins developed for snakes endemic to the same hemisphere [3]. A randomized, placebo-controlled and blinded study affirmed the ability of a Mexican *Micrurus* (coral snake) antivenin and an Australian *Notechis* (tiger snake) antivenin to prevent lethality from United States *Micrurus fulvius fulvius* venom in a mouse model [4].

Snakes—Viperidae (retractable front fangs)

Envenomations by these species are generally treated with volume support and antivenin; many cause life-threatening coagulation deficits.

Gaboon viper

Bitis gabonica venom exerts a number of cytotoxic and cardiovascular effects. Cytotoxic effects include widespread hemorrhage caused by the presence of two hemorrhagic proteins. This viper produces prodigious amounts of venom, but the toxicity (weight for weight) is low compared with other poisonous snakes.

Envenomations are characterized by progressive swelling of the affected limb, local necrosis and hemorrhagic edema near the wound, chest tightness, and prolonged coagulation times. Platelet counts are generally not altered.

Saw-scaled viper

Victims envenomated by the northern saw-scaled viper (*Echis sochureki*) develop dramatically prolonged clotting tests and exhibit systemic bleeding. Antivenin made (in part) with *Echis carinatus* venom from southern India has been traditionally relatively ineffective in restoring coagulation to these patients. Intracranial bleeding can occur with possible long-term neurologic sequelae.

Puff adder

The puff adder (*Bitis arietans*) is a highly toxic venomous snake responsible for a large proportion of the venomous snakebites in sub-Saharan Africa. Puff adder envenomation causes tissue necrosis, hypotension, coagulopathy, thrombocytopenia, and spontaneous bleeding. Severe coagulopathy may occur. Veterinarians treating severe cases should be prepared to administer multiple vials of antivenin.

Snakes—Crotalidae (retractable front fangs)

Pit vipers

North American pit viper antivenins (ACP, Polyvalent Equine-Origin Antivenin [Crotalidae], Fort Dodge Laboratories, Ames, Iowa; CroFab,

Crotalidae Polyvalent Immune Fab Ovine, Protherics, Brentwood, Tennessee) have shown cross-reactivity with fractions of most of the New World pit viper venoms. When a specific antivenin for an exotic pit viper is not available, it would be reasonable (in the author's opinion) to administer them.

Fer-de-lance

Bothrops asper venom induces complex local effects such as myonecrosis, edema, and especially hemorrhage. North American pit viper antivenin (ACP) is highly effective because *Bothrops asper* is one of the immunizing snakes in Fort Dodge's veterinary pit viper antivenin.

Green pit viper

Green viper (*Trimeresurus albolabris* and *Trimeresurus macrops*) venom has a thrombinlike effect in vitro but causes a defibrination syndrome in vivo. The effects of the venom on the fibrinolytic system have not been well characterized. Fibrinolytic system activation is very common.

South American rattlesnake

The venom of the South American rattlesnake (*Crotalus durissus terrificus*) has mainly hemolytic and neurotoxic pathophysiologic activities. There is also a systemic myotoxic action of the venom characterized by the release of myoglobin from damaged skeletal muscle into serum and urine. Some victims develop acute renal failure secondarily. This snake is also an immunizing venom for the North American pit viper antivenin produced by Fort Dodge laboratories (ACP).

Palm viper

A myotoxic phospholipase A2 has been isolated from the venom of the arboreal snake *Bothriechis schlegelii* (formerly *Bothrops schlegelii*) from Costa Rica. The toxin induces rapid myonecrosis on intramuscular injection in mice [5]. *Bothriechis schlegelii* venom is considered to have no hemorrhagic activity.

Snakes—Colubridae (rear fangs)

Rear-fanged snakes, in general, have a poor venom delivery system that may prevent some species from being more medically significant. Bites in which the snake gets a deep grip and remains attached for a longer period of time increase the snake's ability to deliver a larger venom load to the victim. There are several colubrids capable of significant envenomations (Box 1).

Boomslang

The boomslang (*Dispholidus typus*) from sub-Saharan Africa is a slender arboreal snake that can grow to over 2 m in length. The boomslang venom is a potent procoagulant, causing a consumption coagulopathy with resultant

---

Box 1. Colubrids capable of significant envenomation

Capable of fatal envenoming
  Dispholidus typus (boomslang)
  Thelortornis spp (vine, twig, or bird snakes)

Capable of severe envenoming
  Malpolon monspessulanus (Montpellier snake)

---

profuse hemorrhage. The only effective treatment is the administration of specific antiserum; however, administration of fresh blood and plasma appears to be the most useful supportive measure. Despite a fully established clinical picture of diffuse intravascular coagulation, response to specific boomslang antivenin is usually immediate, even administered as late as 86 hours after the bite.

Lizards

Gila monster

Only two species of lizards in the world are poisonous: the North and Central American *Heloderma* spp—the Mexican beaded lizard and, more famously, the Gila monster. The venom from these lizards is used for defense only and not for capture of prey. These lizards have a poorly developed venom delivery system and must chew on their victim, allowing the wound to be bathed in the venom.

The venom contains multiple fractions, including hyaluronidase (spreading factor), arginine hydrolase (thought to have a bradykinin releasing–like activity), kallikrein-like enzymes (which cause vasodilatation, increased capillary permeability, edema, activation of extravascular smooth muscle, and pain), and phospholipase (uncouples oxidative phosphorylation and releases histamine, kinin, serotonin, acetylcholine, and slow-reacting substance). Gilatoxin is a neurotoxic protein.

Clinical signs include weakness, nausea, muscle fasciculations, polyuria, salivation, tachycardia, and hypotension. Aphonia has been described in cats. Numerous broken teeth may be in the bite wound.

Treatment consists of intravenous fluids to control hypotension and pain management. The wound may be irrigated with lidocaine and gently probed for broken lizard teeth.

Arthropods

Spiders

There are several medically significant spider genera capable of inducing clinical manifestations in mammals (Box 2).

Box 2. Clinically important spider genera

Loxosceles
Latrodectus
Tegenaria
Phoneutria
Atrax

Widow spiders

Widow spiders of the genus *Latrodectus* have worldwide distribution (Box 3). The black widow spider is found in North America, with the female of the species being medically important. Although there are a variety of these spiders, the venom is antigenically similar. The spider can control the amount of venom injected; approximately 15% of black widow spider bites are "dry," with no venom injected.

There are five or six biologically active proteins in the venom. Most important is the potent neurotoxin α-latrotoxin, which induces neurotransmitter release from nerve terminals. This toxin allows the formation of a channel for monovalent cation exchange, which is then functionally locked open. This depolarization promotes calcium-independent release of the neurotransmitters acetylcholine and norepinephrine (and others) down concentration gradients and inhibits their subsequent reuptake. Acetylcholine, noradrenaline, dopamine, glutamate, and enkephalin systems are all susceptible to the toxin.

Box 3. Widow spiders

North America
 Latrodectus mactans mactans (black widow)
 Latrodectus geometricus (brown widow)
 Latrodectus bishopi (red-legged widow)
 Latrodectus variolus
 Latrodectus hesperus (western black widow)

Australia, New Zealand
 Latrodectus mactans hasselti (red-backed spider)

Europe, South America
 Latrodectus tredecimguttatus (Kara Kurt (black wolf))

Asia, Middle East
 Latrodectus pallidus

Africa
 Latrodectus indistinctus (black button spider)

Clinical signs are minimal locally. In dogs, systemic manifestation of the envenomation syndrome includes regional numbness, tenderness in draining lymph nodes, hyperesthesia, progressive muscle pain, and fasciculations in the affected region. Cramping of the large muscle masses is common; abdominal rigidity without tenderness is a hallmark clinical sign; progression to paralysis is possible. Systemic hypertension and tachycardia should be anticipated. Death is usually due to respiratory or cardiovascular collapse.

Cats are extremely sensitive to this spider toxin, and death is common. Paralytic signs may appear early in the syndrome. Severe pain is exhibited by loud vocalizations and howling. The cat often has excessive salivation and restlessness; vomiting and diarrhea are common. Also seen are muscular tremors, cramping, and ataxia before the onset of paralysis. Hypertension and tachycardia are common. The author has had four cats vomit the spider onto the examination table.

Treatment relies on the administration of *Latrodectus* antivenin. Worldwide, several antivenin products have been developed. In the United States, the primary antivenin is equine-origin (*Latrodectus*) Lyovac antivenin (Merck Sharp & Dohme, Whitehouse Station, New Jersey). This antivenin is produced using old technologies, and the equine-based product has a significant amount of protein impurities. A Mexican biologics company has a purified equine Fab2 antivenin (Polyvalent Latrodectus Anti-spider Fabotherapic, Laboratorios Bioclone, Col. Toriello Guerra, Tlalpan, México) that is in clinical trials in Arizona. One vial of either antivenin is the common treatment dose, and clinical response is rapid, usually within 30 minutes. Newer antivenins have no extraneous proteins and decreased chances of allergic reactions.

Brown spiders

Brown spiders (*Loxosceles* spp) have a worldwide distribution. They are known in the United States as the brown recluse or violin spider (*Loxosceles reclusa*). There are 13 species of brown spiders in North America. *Loxosceles laeta* and *Loxosceles gaucho* are indigenous to South America. *Loxosceles rufescens* is the Mediterranean variety.

The venom has eight major and four minor electrophoritic bands. The primary venom dermonecrotic protein is sphingomyelinase D (also known as phospholipase D). This protein binds to the cellular membrane and chemotactically pulls in polymorphonuclear leukocytes. The venom induces coagulation and occlusion of small capillaries, leading to marked tissue necrosis. When the sphingomyelinase D interacts with C-reactive protein and calcium, there is a direct hemolytic effect. The venom also acts on lipids, freeing fragments into circulation that act as emboli and as inflammatory mediators; therefore, bites to fatty areas can develop more severe local tissue destruction.

Clinical signs include local irritation and soreness. A classic "bull's-eye lesion" may develop over multiple hours, with a dark eschar in an ischemic zone surrounded by a hyperemic background. Over the next 2 weeks, the lesion can mature into a necrotic indolent ulcer that can persist for months. Systemic clinical signs can rarely occur with the onset of a hemolytic crisis (usually with in 24 hours). Hemoglobinuria can induce renal failure. Disseminated intravascular coagulation and thrombocytopenia are possible sequelae.

There is no antidote; however, several countries are developing antivenins. Treatment is supportive and may include the use of dapsone.

Scorpions

Several species of scorpions can be found in pet stores, most commonly the emperor scorpion (*Pandinus imperator*), the Flat Rocks scorpion (*Hadogenes* sp), and the Asian forest scorpion (*Heterometus* sp). All of these have weak venom and are considered harmless. It should be noted, however, that any foreign protein can induce anaphylactic allergic reactions in sensitive individuals.

Most scorpions of greatest concern belong to the family Buthidae; in addition, there is a single dangerous genus in the families Scorpionidae and Diplocentridae (Box 4). A general rule is scorpions with big pincers and small, thin tails usually have less toxic venom, whereas species with very small or delicate pincers and big, fat tails are to be viewed as potentially very dangerous.

Scorpion antivenin is generally species specific and needs to be administered within the first couple of hours post envenomation. Although it may be available at a local zoo, the timeline from envenomation to diagnosis and treatment usually precludes the use of scorpion antivenin.

The red scorpion

The red scorpion (*Mesobuthus tamulus*) from India is regarded as their most dangerous. Envenomation causes local pain, and systemic toxicity is

---

Box 4. Family and genus of medically significant scorpions

Buthidae
  Buthus
  Androctonus
  Leiurus
  Centruroides
  Tityus
  Parabuthus
  Mesobuthus

Scorpionidae
  Hemiscorpion

Diplocentridae
  Nebo

induced by the massive release of catecholamines, leading to severe cardio-pulmonary toxicity. Mortality rates as high as 30% were recorded in humans in the 1960s. These rates have dropped to around 3% with the use of calcium channel blockers and vasodilators [6].

The black scorpion

Black scorpion (*Androctonus crassicauda*) venom triggers a cholinergic response so that victims develop increased urination, incontinence, increased gastrointestinal motility, and exocrine gland hypersecretions. To a lesser extent, neurologic signs can develop, including confusion, restlessness, coma, seizures, paralysis, and muscle spasms in the area of the bite site.

Hemiscorpion lepturus

Hemiscorpion lepturus does not have a neurotoxin but contains potent cytotoxic venom. The sting site in humans is initially a bluish lesion, followed by a red halo effect. It can progress to a sloughing, necrotic wound. This venom has caused hemolysis and renal failure. In severe envenomations, cardiovascular toxicity can occur.

Five-keeled gold scorpion

The Middle Eastern five-keeled gold scorpion (*Leiurus quinquestriatus*) is also known as the death stalker because of its 18% death rate in children [7]. The initial clinical signs are intense local pain, redness, and edema. Next, a massive release of acetylcholine and catecholamines occurs, resulting in severe hypertension, tachyarrhythmias, and pulmonary edema. Parasympathomimetic signs can follow with bradycardia and heart block. Cardiac damage can occur. Pancreatitis, hypersalivation, convulsions, agitation, and priapism have all been documented in envenomated humans.

Yellow scorpion

Androctonus australis is a yellow scorpion from North Africa. Envenomations by this species are classified into three grades in humans Table 1.

Fat-tailed scorpion

Parabuthus spp can induce neuromuscular toxicity without a significant autonomic system response.

Table 1
Envenomation grades for North African scorpions

Grade	Clinical syndrome
1	Local sings only, intense pain, paresthesias, irritability
2	Grade 1 signs plus restlessness, tachycardia, moderate hyperthermia, and increased cholinergic tone leading to hypersalivation, rhinorrhea, vomiting, and diarrhea
3	Cardiocirculatory shock, respiratory failure, pulmonary edema, hyperthermia, seizures, hyperglycemia, depressed level of consciousness

Brazilian yellow scorpion

Severe *Tityus* sp envenomations can induce restlessness, tachypnea, vomiting, shock, seizures, and inflammation of the myocardium. There is a remarkable incidence of acute pancreatitis in human victims (and experimentally in dogs, but at a larger venom dose) [8,9].

Bark scorpion

Centruroides spp are small yellow scorpions and the primary scorpions of importance in Mexico and in the state of Arizona. From 1940 to 1960, over tenfold more deaths occurred in Mexico due to scorpion envenomations than from all venomous snakebites. Respiratory failure is the usual cause of death. Human victims are hyperexcitable, restless, tachycardic or bradycardic, and nauseated; have gastric distention, vomiting, diarrhea, excessive lacrimation; exhibit nystagmus (roving eye movements) and dysphasia; and usually have hypertension (hypotension can occur), heart failure, convulsions, and ataxia. The envenomation syndrome can mature to a comatose state.

Treatment for most victims demonstrating only local signs is primarily observation and symptomatic therapy (for pain management). Victims severely affected should be hospitalized. Airway management is key, and cardiovascular and respiratory systems should be closely monitored.

Although there are many treatments for scorpion envenomation, few have been rigorously tested for their validity. One of the few treatments subjected to randomized, controlled, and blinded human study was anti-inflammatory corticosteroids, which showed no benefit [10]. Digoxin, diuretics, antihistamines, dopamine, dobutamine, and β-adrenergic blockers are not recommended.

Care should be taken if atropine is used to attempt control of excessive cholinergic clinical signs. Although atropine may be of benefit for bradycardia and can decrease airway secretions, it can worsen tachycardia and hypertension. Parasympathetic effects are usually transient; however, the risk of aspiration can be high. The attending veterinarian must decide the atropine risk-to-benefit ratio for each case.

Vasodilator therapy may be of some benefit in controlling cardiopulmonary effects of the venom, but no controlled studies have been performed. Captopril could potentially worsen pulmonary edema. Nitroprusside may benefit patients that have life-threatening pulmonary edema. Nonsteroidal anti-inflammatory drugs, quinine, aminophylline, and dantrolene potentially have some benefit as adjunct therapies.

Amphibians

Toads

Toad (*Bufo* spp) toxicity is varied, with the most toxic poison produced by the cane or marine toad (*Bufo marinus*). The toxin is secreted from the toad's large parotid glands and rapidly absorbed across the mucus membranes into the victim's circulation. A wide variety of biologically active compounds are present in toad toxin: dopamine, epinephrine, norepinephrine, serotonin, bufotenine, bufagenins, bufotoxins, and indolealkylamines. Bufagenins and bufotoxins are cardioactive digitalislike substances.

First clinical signs are pawing at the mouth, brick red gums, hypersalivation, vocalization, and "foaming at the mouth." The patient is often disoriented and stuporous. Severe toxicosis leads to convulsions and coma. Risk of cardiac arrhythmias is high.

Initial treatment is to copiously flush the mouth of the victim while trying to keep the patient from swallowing the rinsing liquid. Seizures should be controlled, then cardiac status, with rate and rhythm, should be immediately assessed by ECG.

Bradycardic or heart block patients can be treated with atropine, which may have the added benefit of decreasing salivation. Atropine is not a true antidote, and if the patient has tachycardia, its use is contraindicated. Tachycardia can be treated with propranolol; ventricular tachycardia with lidocaine.

If the clinical syndrome is severe, digoxin Fab (DIGIBIND, Digoxin Immune Fab [Ovine], GlaxoSmithKlien, Pharma, Italy) may bind the digoxinlike components of the toxin. Hyperthermia is often a sequela of the intense muscular activity of the patient, and the clinician should monitor for its presence.

Frogs

Poison arrow frogs (Dendrobatidae) are small, colorful frogs that inhabit the jungles of South America and can be purchased at many pet stores. The skin secretes a poisonous mixture of complex alkaloids, the most potent of which is batrachotoxin. One species, *Phyllobates terribilis*, contains 500 μg of batrachotoxin per frog. Pumiliotoxin, epibatidin, and histrionicotoxin are among the other toxins in the complex alkaloid mixture.

Batrachotoxin blocks sodium channels from closing after depolarization, so the nerve continuously fires, which can lead to cardiac arrest. Pumiliotoxin is a hydroquinoline. Histrionicotoxin has a high affinity for the ion channel of the acetylcholine receptor. When bred in captivity, these frogs lack these toxins unless fed foods containing the precursors for the toxins. The primary venom precursors come from ingested ants, beetles, and millipedes. Treatment is largely supportive.

Salamanders and newts (Salimandridae)

Salamanders (*Salamandra* spp) store toxins in the parotid glands on either side of the neck, just behind the head. The toxins in salamander parotid secretions are the steroidal alkaloids samandarine and samandaridine. These compounds act centrally, inducing seizures. Treatment consists of seizure control and supportive care.

Newt (*Notophtalmus* sp) toxin is a tetrodotoxin that seems to be synthesized by bacteria. Newts that are captive bred do not have this bacterial flora and therefore have no tetrodotoxin. Tetrodotoxin blocks sodium channels on the excitable membranes. Victims can be fully conscious but unable to move, with a complete flaccid paralysis. Treatment consists of supportive care and possibly hydroxyzine.

References

[1] Laothong C, Sitprija V. Decreased parasympathetic activities in Malayan krait (*Bungarus candidus*) envenoming. Toxicon 2001;39(9):1353–7.

[2] Kularatne SA. Common krait (*Bungarus caeruleus*) bite in Anuradhapura, Sri Lanka: a prospective clinical study, 1996–98. Postgrad Med J 2002;78(919):276–80.

[3] de Roodt AR, Paniagua-Solis JF, Dolab JA, et al. Effectiveness of two common antivenoms for North, Central, and South American *Micrurus* envenomations. J Toxicol Clin Toxicol 2004;42(2):171–8.

[4] Wisniewski MS, Hill RE, Havey JM, et al. Australian tiger snake (*Notechis scutatus*) and Mexican coral snake (Micruris species) antivenoms prevent death from United States coral snake (*Micrurus fulvius fulvius*) venom in a mouse model. J Toxicol Clin Toxicol 2003;41(1): 7–10.

[5] Angulo Y, Chaves E, Alape A, et al. Isolation and characterization of a myotoxic phospholipase A2 from the venom of the arboreal snake *Bothriechis* (Bothrops) *schlegelii* from Costa Rica. Arch Biochem Biophys 1997;339(2):260–6.

[6] Bawaskar HS, Bawaskar PH. Treatment of envenoming by Mesobuthus tamulus (Indian red scorpion). Trans R Soc Trop Med Hyg 1992;86(4):459.

[7] Dudin AA, Rambaud-Cousson A, Thalji A, et al. Scorpion sting in children in the Jerusalem area: a review of 54 cases. Ann Trop Paediatr 1991;11(3):217–23.

[8] Bartholomew C. Acute scorpion pancreatitis in Trinidad. Br Med J 1970;1(5697):666–8.

[9] George Angus LD, Salzman S, Fritz K, et al. Chronic relapsing pancreatitis from a scorpion sting in Trinidad. Ann Trop Paediatr 1995;15(4):285–9.

[10] Abroug F, Nouira S, Haguiga H, et al. High-dose hydrocortisone hemisuccinate in scorpion envenomation. Ann Emerg Med 1997;30(1):23–7.

ELSEVIER
SAUNDERS

VETERINARY
CLINICS
Exotic Animal Practice

Vet Clin Exot Anim 11 (2008) 389–401

Toxicologic Information Resources for Reptile Envenomations

Jude McNally, RPh, DABAT*, Keith Boesen, PharmD,
Leslie Boyer, MD, FACMT

*Arizona Poison and Drug Information Center, College of Pharmacy, University of Arizona,
1295 N. Martin, Room B308, Tucson, AZ 85721, USA*

The United States is the largest importer of reptiles in the world with an estimated 1.5 to 2.0 million households keeping one or more reptiles. Snakes account for about 11% of these imports and it has been estimated that as many as 9% of these reptiles are venomous [1]. Envenomations by nonindigenous venomous species are a rare but often serious medical emergency. These bites are likely to occur in two distinctly different communities in the United States. Bites may occur during the care and handling of legitimate collections found in universities, zoos, or museums. Maintenance of these animals inherently places curators and zoo veterinarians at some risk. The other predominant source of exotic envenomation is from amateur collectors participating in importation, propagation, and trade of non-native species. This latter group is sometimes referred to as the "underground zoo" [2]. State laws vary on the legality of keeping exotic venomous species, but in this age of worldwide Internet access, illegal trade can occur without accountability. It is reasonable to assume that exotic venomous species can be found throughout the United States. It is further reasonable to expect that the amateur herpetoculturists will at some time seek veterinary care for their valuable collection.

The Toxic Exposure Surveillance System (TESS) is a database of poison center calls compiled from data submitted from over 60 poison centers across the country. Reporting bias prevents these data from being an accurate account of actual poison exposure; however, with the addition of more than 2 million cases each year it is the largest database of its kind and may accurately reflect trends in specific exposures such as snakebite. Evaluation of the 3 most recent years of published data, 2003 through 2005, shows that

* Corresponding author.
E-mail address: mcnally@pharmacy.arizona.edu (J. McNally).

rattlesnake bites account for the majority of known reported venomous snakebites averaging 1226 bites per year. Copperhead bites are second averaging 1048 bites year and cottonmouth snakes are third with an average of 187 reported annually. Most notably, exotic venomous snakebites come in fourth, averaging 118 per year. The number of exotic venomous snakebites has surpassed the indigenous coral snakebites, which average only 85 bites per year (Table 1) [3–5].

The actual risk of dying from snakebite in the United States is quite low [6]. It is worth noting, however, that there is a higher death rate reported from venomous exotic snakebites than from all the other indigenous categories described in Table 1. Between 2003 and 2005 TESS reported two exotic snakebite deaths from a total of 355 bites (0.85% fatality rate). During this same period there were six deaths from a total of 3678 rattlesnake bites (0.16% fatality rate) and three from a total of 1241 unknown Crotaline bites (0.24% fatality rate). No deaths were reported from coral snakes, copperheads, or cottonmouths during this 3-year period. The combined fatality rate for all indigenous venomous snakebites reported in TESS is 0.10%, less than an eighth the fatality rate for non-native snakebite occurring in the United States [3–5].

Outside the United States, snakebites are a significant cause of morbidity and mortality. Conservative estimates of greater than 100,000 deaths annually are frequently sited [7]. Fatality rates exceeding 50% have been described in some parts of the world. The extent to which this high mortality rate is driven by more acutely toxic snake species versus the lack of modern medical care is not known [8].

There are approximately 2700 different snake species in the world and of these about one fifth are venomous. The venomous snakes can be found in four different families: Atractaspididae, Colubridae, Elapidae, and Viperidae. In the United States, medical practitioners concern themselves primarily with bites from the Viperidae subfamily Crotalinae and with a single genus of the Elapidae family, *Micrurus*. The Elapidae family is divided into three subfamilies that include highly toxic members such as the cobras,

Table 1
Snakebites reported to TESS 2003 through 2005

Snake	2003	2004	2005
Copperhead	997	1098	1051
Coral	97	99	58
Cottonmouth	175	192	194
Crotaline: unknown	397	431	413
Rattlesnake	1245	1178	1255
Venomous exotic snake	126	131	98
Nonvenomous exotic snake	138	131	42
Unknown exotic	9	2	6
Nonvenomous snake	1818	1803	1552
Unknown snake	1887	2147	1972

mambas, and kraits, none of which are native to the United States. The only Elapids indigenous to the United States are the coral snakes including the genera *Micrurus* and *Micruroides*. The subfamily Crotalinae includes the genera *Crotalus* and *Agkistrodon*. Snakes in this subfamily include rattlesnakes, copperheads, and cottonmouths. These are the snakes that most US clinicians experience in treating envenomations. The Atractaspididae is the most recently recognized family of venomous snakes commonly referred to as stiletto snakes. Colubridae is the largest family consisting of both venomous and nonvenomous snakes. The African boomslang is one of the most notorious members of this family [9].

It is widely accepted that the mainstay of medical management of envenomation by a US snake species is antivenom. A polyvalent crotaline antibody antivenom, CroFab (Protherics, Nashville TN) has been developed to treat envenomations from all the native Crotalines [10]. CroFab is the only US Food and Drug Administration (FDA)-approved antivenom still being manufactured. Fort Dodge manufactures a Whole IgG antibody against Crotalinae venom approved for veterinary use only. Antivenoms are also occasionally used in the management of *Latrodectus* species (black widow spiders) and *Centruroides* species (bark scorpions) envenomations. There has been a historic reluctance to use the scorpion and spider antivenoms as first-line therapy because of the high incidence of hypersensitivity reactions and the relative safety and efficacy of palliative management [11,12]. Newer Fab2 antivenoms against *Latrodectus* and *Centruroides* species are currently in clinical trials.

In the case of snakebite, the complexity and severity of the clinical manifestations frequently warrant a relatively lower threshold for deciding to treat with antivenom. This may be especially true when managing an exotic snakebite because of the potential severity of symptoms refractory to palliative care [10].

At present, the only antivenoms approved by the FDA for sale and distribution within the United States are those indicated for the treatment of bites and stings by animals native to the United States (pit vipers, coral snakes, and black widow spiders). When people in the United States are bitten by non-native species, there is no governmental or commercial system for the timely acquisition of foreign-manufactured antivenoms. Because of the small number of cases in the United States, there is not sufficient economic incentive for pharmaceutical companies to manufacture or import these exotic antivenoms. There is, however, a special provision within FDA regulations that allows zoos exclusively to order and stock foreign-manufactured, non-FDA–approved exotic antivenoms for protection of zoo staff in the event of an emergency.

The Antivenom Index (AI) is a compilation of information related to these stores of antivenom from zoos across the country. The AI is the product of a cooperative effort between the American Association of Poison Control Centers (AAPCC) and the American Zoo Association (AZA). For over 20 years the AI existed in a paper form that was inevitably out

---

Box 1. Selected references pertaining to *Bitis* species

Bey TA, Boyer LV, Walter FG, et al. Exotic snakebite: envenomation by an African puff adder (*Bitis arietans*). J Emerg Med 1997;15(6):827–31.

Blaylock R. Epidemiology of snakebite in Eshowe, KwaZulu-Natal, South Africa. Toxicon 2004;43:159–66.

Britt A, Burkhart K. *Naja naja* cobra bite. Am J Emerg Med 1997;15:529–31.

Egan VT. African puff adders *Bitis arietans*. Reptile & Amphibian Magazine 1996(May/June):26–32.

Harrison RA, Oliver J, Hasson SS, et al. Novel sequences encoding venom C-type lectins are conserved in phylogenetically and geographically distince *Echis* and *Bitis* viper species. Gene 2003;315:95–102.

Lavonas EJ, Tomaszewski CA, Ford MD, et al. Severe puff adder (*Bitis arietans*) envenomation with coagulopathy. J Toxicol Clin Toxicol 2002;40(7):911–8.

Marsh NA, Whaler BC. The Gaboon viper (*Bitis gabonica*): its biology, venom components and toxinology. Toxicon 1984;22(5):669–94.

Marsh N, Gattullo D, Pagliaro P, et al. The gaboon viper, *Bitis gabonica*: hemorrhagic, metabolic, cardiovascular and clinical effects of the venom. Life Sci 1997;61(8):763–9.

McNally T, Conway GS, Jackson L, et al. Accidental envenoming by a gobbon viper (*Bitis gabonica*): the haemostatic disturbances observed and investigation of in vitro haemostatic properties of whole venom. Trans Royal Soc Trop Med Hyg 1993;87:66–70.

Spawls S, Branch B. *The dangerous snakes of Africa*. Sanibel Island (FL): Ralph Curtis Books; 1995.

---

dated as soon as it was published. It was updated to an electronic form in 2006. The AI currently exists as a limited access, Web-based program run by the AZA. It is a relational database made up of tables including a list of common and scientific names of venomous animals; member institution location and emergency contact information; poison control center location and contact information; antivenom indications for specific species; species information for antivenoms; available inventories of specific antivenoms; available antivenom product by name, quantity, and cost from manufacturers; manufacturer's location and contact information; and other necessary notes regarding acquisition of antivenoms. The AI currently lists over 1500 scientific names of venomous animals from 35 different countries and 55 manufacturers of antivenoms.

Box 2. Selected references pertaining to *Bothrops* species

Avila-Aguero ML, Valverde K, Gutierrez J, et al. Venomous snake bites in children and adolescents: a 12 year retrospective review. Venom Anim Toxins 2001;7:69–84.

Battellino C, Piazza R, da Silva AMM, et al. (2003). Assessment of efficacy of bothropic antivenom therapy on microcirculatory effects induced by *Bothrops jararaca* snake venom. Toxicon 2003;41:583–93.

Bauab FA, Junqueira GR, Morato Corradini MC, et al. Clinical and epidemiologic aspects of the 'urutu' lance-headed viper (*Bothrops alternatus*) bite in a Brazilian hospital. Trop Med Parasitol 1994;45:243–5.

Benvenuti LA, Franca FOS, Barbaro DC, et al. Pulmonary hemorrhage causing rapid death after *Bothrops juraracussu* snakebite: a case report. Toxicon 2003;42:331–4.

Bucher B, Canonge D, Thomas B, et al. Clinical indicators of envenoming and serum levels of venom antigens in patients bitten by *Bothrops lanceolatus* in Martinique. Trans Royal Soc Trop Med Hyg 1997;91:186–90.

Franca FOS, Barbaro KC, Fan HW, et al. Envenoming by *Bothrops jararaca* in Brazil: association between venom antigenemia and severity of admission to hospital. Trans Royal Soc Trop Med Hyg 2003;97:312–7.

Milani Jr. R, Jorge MT, Ferraz De Campos FP, et al. Snake bites by the jararacussu (*Bothrops jarraracussu*): clinicopathological studies of 29 proven cases in Sao Paulo, Brazil. Q J Med 1997;90:323–34.

Nishioka SDA, Silveira PVP. A clinical and epidemiologic study of 292 cases of lance-headed viper bite in a Brazilian teaching hospital. Am J Trop Med Hyg 1992;47:805–10.

Pardal PP de O, Souza SM, Monteiro da C de C, et al. Clinical trial of two antivenoms for the treatment of *Bothrops* and *Lachesis* bites in the northeastern Amazon region of Brazil. Trans Roy Soc Trop Med Hyg 2004;98(1):28–42.

Pinho FMO, Burdmann E de Almeida. Fatal cerebral hemorrhage and acute renal failure after young *Bothrops jararacussu* snake bite. Renal Failure 2001;23:269–77.

Russell FE, Walter FG, Bey TA, et al. (1997) Snakes and snakebite in Central America (Review article). Toxicon 1997;35:1469–522.

Saravia P, Rojas E, Escalante T, et al. The venom of *Bothrops
asper* from Guatemala: toxic activities and neutralization
by antivenoms. Toxicon 2001;39:401–5.
Thomas L, Chausson N, Uzan J, et al. Thrombotic stroke
following snake bites by the "Fer-de-Lance" *Bothrops
lanceolatus* in Marinique despite antivenom treatment: a report
of three cases. Toxicon 2006;48:23–8.

Each of the 55 AZA institutions participating in the AI is responsible for updating the institution's inventory and personnel information as changes occur. Each participating institution has the ability to view the other institutions' antivenom inventories, but changes to the AI index can only be made to their own institution's profile. All AAPCC member poison centers have read-only access to the AI database. When a poison center is contacted regarding an exotic snakebite, they are able to cross reference common names with scientific names to select appropriate foreign antivenoms. They are further able to locate the closest zoo stocking that antivenom and identify the designated zoo contact. The poison specialist is also able to access the actual number of vials available and the expiration dates of those vials. Poison centers are part of a nationwide toll-free network: dialing (800) 222-1222 will connect the caller with the closest certified regional poison center.

Whenever a snake envenomation happens, time is of the essence [10]. This may be particularly true with envenomations by many of the non-native species. Anyone working with exotic snakes should assume a bite is at least possible if not probable and should have an advance written plan of action to avoid time delays when an incident happens. Development of this plan should include discussions with regional poison centers and local hospitals to alert them to the possibility they may be requested to treat an exotic bite. Most health care providers are inexperienced with the manifestations and management of exotic snakebites. Sharing in advance your written plan may hasten clinical decisions. The plan should include details such as patient transportation, identifying which specific antivenoms would be most efficacious, and instructions for rapid acquisition of the antivenom. Identification of appropriate antivenoms can be done through a regional poison center in advance of a bite; however, the closest location of the antivenom and the amount in stock are subject to change at any time. At the time of an actual bite, the poison center should still be contacted immediately to request the most updated information. Seifert and colleagues [13] have developed a position statement regarding institutions housing venomous reptiles. This brief document describes all the essential elements to consider in preparing your advance plan.

A treatment guideline should also be developed for each species held. The guideline should be developed after a thorough review of the medical

Box 3. Selected references pertaining to cobra species

Al-Asmari AK, Al-Abdulaa IH, Crouch RG, et al. Assessment of an ovine antivenom raised against venom from the desert black cobra (*Walterinnesia aegyptia*). Toxicon 1997;35(1):141–5.

Blaylock RS, Lichtman AR, Potgeiter PD. Clinical manifestations of Cape cobra (*Naja nivea*) bites. S Afr Med J 1985;68:342–4.

Britt A, Burkhart K. *Naja naja* cobra bite. Am J Emerg Med 1997;15:529–31.

Gold BS. Neostigmine for the treatment of neurotoxicity following envenomation by the Asiatic cobra. Ann Emerg Med 1996;28(1):87–9.

Gold BS, Pyle P. Successful treatment of neurotoxic king cobra envenomation in Myrtle Beach, South Carolina. Ann Emerg Med 1998;32(6):736–8.

Homma C, Tu AT. Antivenom for the treatment of local tissue damage due to envenomation by Southeast Asian snakes. Ineffectiveness in the prevention of local tissue damage in mice after envenomation. Am J Trop Med Hyg 1970;19:880–4.

Hung D-Z, Liau M-Y, Lin-Shiau S-Y. The clinical significance of venom detection in patients of cobra snakebite. Toxicon 2003;41:409–15.

Kasilo OMJ, Nhachi CFB. A retrospective study of poisoning due to snake venom in Zimbabwe. Hum Exp Toxicol 1993;12:15–8.

Kulkarnia ML, Anees S. Snake venom poisoning: experience with 633 cases. Indian Pediatr 1994;31(10):1239–43.

Mitrakul C, Dhamkrong-At A, Futrakul P, et al. Clinical features of neurotoxic snake bite and resonse to antivenom in 47 children. Am J Trop Med Hyg 1984;33(6):1258–66.

Pochanugool C, Limthongkul S, Wilde H. Management of Thai cobra bites with a single bolus of antivenin. Wilderness Environ Med 1997;8:20–3.

Theakston RDG, Phillips RE, Warrell DA, et al. Envenoming by the common krait (*Bugarus caeruleus*) and Sri Lankan cobra (*Naja naja naja*): efficacy and complications of therapy with Haffkine antivenom. Trans Roy Soc Trop Med Hyg 1990;84:301–8.

Tilbury CR. Observations on the bite of the Mozambique spitting cobra (*Naja mossambica mossambica*). SA Med J 1982;61:308–13.

Warrell DA. Clinical toxicology of snakebite in Africa and the Middle East and Asia. In: Meier J, White J, editors. Clinical toxicology of animal venoms and poisons. Boca Raton (FL): CRC Press; 1995. p. 433–594.

Warrell DA, Ormerod LD. Snake venom ophthalmia and blindness caused by the spitting cobra (*Naja nigricollis*) in Nigeria. Am J Trop Med Hyg 1976;25(3):525–9.

Watt G, Padre L, Tuazon L, et al. Bites by the Philippine cobra (*Naja naja philippinensis*): prominent neurotoxicity with minimal local signs. Am J Trop Med Hyg 1988;39(3):306–11.

Box 4. Selected references pertaining to *Echis* species

Bawaskar HS, Bawaskar PH. Profile of snakebite envenoming in western Maharashtra, India. Trans Roy Soc Trop Med Hyg, 2002;96:79–84.

Benbassat J, Shalev O. Envenomation by *Echis coloratus* (Mideast saw–scaled viper): a review of the literature and indications for treatment. Isr J Med Sci 1993;29:239–50.

Chippaux JP, Lang J, Eddine SA, et al. Clinical safety of a polyvalent F(ab')2 equine antivenom in 233 African snake envenomations: a field trial in Cameroon. Trans Roy Soc Trop Med Hyg 1998;92:657–62.

Gillissen A, Theakston RDG, Barth J, et al. Neurotoxicity, haemostatic disturbances and hemolytic anemia after a bite by a Tunisian saw–scaled or carpet viper (*Echis 'pyramidum'*-complex). Toxicon 1994;32:937–44.

Habib AG, Gebi UI, Onyemelukwe GC. Snake bite in Nigeria. Afr J Med Med Sci 2001;30:171–8.

Meyer WP, Habib AG, Onayade A, et al. First clinical experiences with a new ovine Fab *Echis ocellatus* snake bite antivenom in Nigreria: randomized comparative trial with institute Pasteur serum (Ipser) Africa antivenom. Am J Trop Med Hyg 1997;56(3):291–300.

Punde DP. Management of snake-bite in rural Maharashtra: A 10-year experience. Nat Med J India 2005;18(2):71–5.

Vijeth SR, Dutta TK, Shahapurkar J, Sahai A. Dose and frequency of anti-snake venom injection in treatment of *Echis carinatus* (saw-scaled viper) bite. JAPI 2000;48:187–91.

Warrell DA, Warrell MJ, Edgar W, et al. Comparison of Pasteur and Behringwerke antivenoms in envenoming by the carpet viper (*Echis carinatus*). Brit Med J 1980;280(6214):607–9.

Weis JR, Whatley RE, Glenn JL, Rodgers GM. Prolonged hypofibrinogenemia and protein C activation after envenoming by *Echis carinatus sochureki*. Am J Trop Med Hyg 1991;44(4):452–60.

---

literature pertaining to bites by the specific species of concern. Primary literature, including case reports, may be most useful, the tertiary literature such as textbooks often lack the details pertinent to a specific species. Package inserts for the antivenoms of interest should be obtained in advance of an emergency and used in the guideline development. Many of these are available through the AI. They will provide reconstitution and dosing information but are often not printed in English. Advance translation of the package insert is crucial.

Box 5. Selected references pertaining to *Lachesis* species

Chippaux JP, Theakston RDG. Epidemiologic studies of snake bite in French Guiana. Ann Top Med Parasitol 1987;81(3):301–4.

Jorge MT, Sano-Martins IS, Tomy SC, et al. Snakebite by the bushmaster (*Lachesis muta*) in Brazil: case report and review of the literature. Toxicon 1997;35(4):545–54.

Pardal PPO, Souze SM, Monteiro MRCC, et al. Clinical trial of two antivenoms for the treatment of *Bothrops* and *Lachesis* bites in the north eastern Amazon region of Brazil. Trans R Soc Trop Med Hyg 2004;98:28–42.

Rosenthal R, Meier J, Koelz A, et al. Intestinal ischemia after bushmaster (*Lachesis muta*) snakebite—a case report. Toxicon 2002;40:217–20.

Weinberg ML, Felicori LF, Bello CA, et al. Biochemical properties of a bushmaster snake venom serine proteinase (LV-Ka) and its kinin releaseing activity evaluated in rat mesenteric arterial rings. J Pharmacol Sci 2004;96:333–42.

A clinical toxicologist or a physician knowledgeable and experienced in the management of envenomations should review the treatment guideline.

Boxes 1–7 list selected references pertaining to commonly held exotic species. These articles may be useful in formulating specific treatment guidelines. The AI was the principal resource in correlating the scientific name with the common name.

Box 1 lists references for *Bitis* species. *Bitis* are members of the Viperidae family found throughout Africa and the Middle East. Commonly held species include: *Bitis arietans* (puff adder), *Bitis gabonica* (gaboon viper), and *Bitis nasicornis* (rhinoceros viper).

Box 2 lists references for *Bothrops* snakes from the Crotalinae subfamily. There are more than 36 species of *Bothrops* and many more subspecies. They have a large geographic range, from southern Mexico through South America. They are commonly referred to as lancehead vipers. Commonly held species include *Bothrops alternatus* (urutu), *Bothrops asper* (terciopelo, barba amarilla) *Bothrops atrox* (common lancehead), *Bothrops jararaca* (jararaca), and *Bothrops lanceolatus* (fer-de-lance, Martinique lancehead).

Box 3 lists references for snakes commonly called cobras. The name cobra is used to describe many different genera (*Naja, Boulengerina, Hemachatus, Ophiophagus, Paranaja, Pseudohaje, Walterinnesia*) and species found in the Elapidae family. Some commonly collected cobras include *Boulengerina* (water cobra), *Hemachatus haemachatus* (Rinkhals cobra), *Naja haje* (Egyptian cobra), *Naja melanoleuca* (forest cobra), *Naja mossambica* (Mozambique cobra), *Naja naja atra* (Chinese cobra), *Naja naja kaouthia* (monocellate or monocled cobra), *Naja mandalayensis* (Burmese spitting

---

Box 6. Selected references pertaining to *Dendroaspis* (mamba) species

Aird SD. Ophidian envenomation strategies and role of purines. Toxicon 2002;40:335–93.

Blaylock RSM. Snake bites at Triangle Hospital January 1975 to June 1981. Central Afr J Med 1982;28:1–10.

Harvey WR. Black mamba envenomation. S Afr Med J 1985;67:960.

Hodgson PS, Davidson TM. Biology and treatment of the mamba snakebite. Wilderness Environ Med 1996;2:133–45.

Lisy O, Jougasaki M, Heublein, et al. Renal actions of synthetic *Dendroaspis* natriuretic peptide. Kid Internat 1999;56:502–8.

Munday SW, Willians SR, Clark RF. Dendrotoxin poisoning in a neurobiochemist. J Toxicol Clin Toxicol 2003;41(2):163–5.

Naidoo DP, Lockhat HS, Naiker IP. Myocardial infarction after probable black mamba envenomation. A case report. S Afr Med J 1987;21:388–9.

Radic A, Duran R, Vellom DC et al. Site of fasciculin interaction with acetylcholinesterase. J Biol Chem 1994;269(15):11233–9.

Saunders CR. Report on a black mamba bite of a medical colleague. Central Afr J Med 1980;26:121–2.

van Asegen F, van Rooyen JM, et al. Putative cardiotoxicity of the venoms of three mamba species. Wilderness Environ Med 1996;2:115–21.

---

cobra), *Naja naja naja* (Indian spectacled cobra), *Naja naja oxiana* (Central Asian cobra), *Naja naja sputatrix* (Southern Indonesian spitting cobra, Javan spitting cobra), *Naja nigricollis* (spitting cobra), *Ophiophagus hannah* (king cobra), and *Walterinnesia aegyptia* (desert black cobra).

Box 4 is a list of references for snakes from the *Echis* genus. These members of the Viperinae subfamily are found in Northern Africa the Middle East and Asia. Commonly held species include *Echis pyramidum or Echis carinatus pyramidum* (saw scale or carpet vipers), *Echis coloratus* (painted saw scale or painted carpet viper), and *Echis ocellatus* (West African carpet viper or ocellated carpet viper).

Box 5 is a brief list of references pertaining to the *Lachesis* genus of the Crotalinae family. *Lachesis* species are commonly called bushmasters. These snakes inhabit tropical rain forests in Central and South America. Species found in a captive collection may include *Lachesis muta* (bushmaster), *Lachesis stenophrys* (bushmaster), and *Lachesis melanocephala* (black-headed bushmaster).

Box 6 lists references pertaining to the genus *Dendroaspis*. Species within this genus of the Elapidae family are commonly referred to as mambas.

Box 7. Selected references pertaining to *Vipera* species

Audebert F, Sorkine M, Bon C. Envenoming by viper bites in France: clinical gradation and biological quantification by ELISA. Toxicon 1992;30(5/6):599–609.

Beer E, Putorti F. Dysphonia, an uncommon symptom of systemic neurotoxic envenomation by *Vipera aspis* bite. Report of two cases. Toxicon 1998;36:697–701.

Ben Abraham R, Winkler E, Eshel G, et al. Snakebite poisoning in children—a call for unified clinical guidelines. Eur J Emerg Med 2001;8:189–192.

Bentur Y, Cahana A. Unusual local complications of *Vipera palaestinae* bite. Toxicon 2003;41:633–5.

Cawrse NH, Inglefield CJ, Hayes C, et al. A snake in the clinical grass: late compartment syndrome in a child bitten by an adder. Br J Plastic Surg 2002;55:434–5.

Chou T-S, Lin T-J, Kuo M-C, et al. Eight cases of acute renal failure from *Vipera russelli formosensis* venom after administration of antivenom. Vet Human Toxicol 2002;44(5):278–82.

De Haro L, Robbe-Vincent A, Saliou B, et al. Unusual neurotoxic envenomations by *Vipera aspis aspis* snakes in France. Hum Exp Toxicol 2002;21:137–45.

Karlson-Stiber C, Persson H, Heath A, et al. First clinical experiences with specific sheep Fab fragments in snake bite. Report of a multicentre study of *Vipera berus* envenoming. J Int Med 1997;241:53–8.

Kjellstrom BT. Acute pancreatitis after snake bite. Acta Chir Scand 1989;155:291–2.

Myiint-Lwin, Warrell DA, Phillips RE, et al. Bites by Russell's viper (*Vipera russelli siamensis*) in Burma: haemostatic, vascular and renal disturbances and response to treatment. Lancet 1985;ii:1259–64.

Phillips RE, Theakston RDG, Warrell DA, et al. Paralysis, rhabdomyolysis and haemolysis caused by bites of Russell's viper (*Vipera russelli*) in Sri Lanka: Failure of Indian (Haffkine) antivenom. Quart J Med New Series 68, 1988;257:691–716.

Radonic V, Budimir D, Bradaric N. Envenomation by the horned viper (*Vipera ammodytes* L.). Mil Med 1997;162(3):179–82.

Spawls S, Branch B. (1995) *The dangerous snakes of Africa.* Ralph Curtis Books; 1995.

> Than T, Hutton RA, Myint-Lwin, et al. Haemostatic disturbances
> in patients bitten by Russell's viper (*Vipera russelli siamensis*)
> in Burma. Brit J Haematol 1988;69:513–20.
> Theakston RDG, Reid HA. Effectiveness of Zagreb antivenom
> against envenoming by the adder, *Vipera berus*. Lancet
> 1976;July 17:121–3.
> Winkler V, Chovers M, Almog S, et al. Decreased serum
> cholesterol level after snake bite (*Vipera palaestinae*) as
> a marker of severity of envenomation. J Lab Clin Med
> 1993;121:774–8.
> Woodhams BJ, Wilson SE, Xin BC, et al. Differences between the
> venoms of two sub-species of Russell's viper: *Vipera russelli
> pulchella* and *Vipera russelli siamensis*. Toxicon 1990;28(4):
> 427–33.

They are native to sub-Saharan Africa. Commonly held mamba species include D*endroaspis polylepis* (black mamba, black-mouthed mamba), *Dendroaspis angusticeps* (common green mamba, eastern green mamba, white-mouthed mamba), *Dendroaspis jamesoni* (Jameson's green mamba, Traills green mamba, western green mamba), and *Dendroaspis viridis* (West African green mamba, western green mamba, Hallowells Green Mamba).

Box 7 lists references for snakes in the Viperidae family and *Vipera* genus. They can be found throughout Europe, Russia, and Asia. Commonly collected species include *Vipera berus* (European adder, common adder), *Vipera aspis* (European asp), *Vipera amodytes* (nose-horned viper, long-nosed viper), *Vipera ursinii* (meadow viper), *Vipera lebetina* (Lebitine viper), and *Vipera xanthina* (coastal viper).

References

[1] Centers for Epidemiology and Animal Health. The Reptile and Amphibian Communities in the United States. Jan 2000, USDA:APHI:VS.
[2] Trestrail JH. The "underground zoo"—the problem of exotic venomous snakes in private possession in the United States. Vet Hum Toxicol 1982;24(Suppl):144–9.
[3] Watson WA, Litovitz TL, Klein-Schwartz W, et al. 2003 annual report of the American Association of Poison Control Centers Toxic Exposure Surveillance System. Am J Emerg Med 2004;22:335–404.
[4] Watson WA, Litovitz TL, Klein-Schwartz W, et al. 2004 annual report of the American Association of Poison Control Centers Toxic Exposure Surveillance System. Am J Emerg Med 2005;23(5):589–666.
[5] Lai MW, Klein-Schwartz W, et al. 2005 Annual Report of the American Association of Poison Control Centers' national poisoning and exposure database. Clin Toxicol (Phila) 2006;44:803–932.

[6] Russell FE. Envenomation and treatment of snakes in the United States. Toxicon 1996; 34(2):151.

[7] Chippaux JP. Snakebites: appraisal of the global situation. Bull World Health Organ 1998; 76(5):515–24.

[8] Currie BJ. Snakebite in tropical Australia: a prospective study in the "Top End" of the Northern Territory. Med J Aust 2004;181(11–12):693–7.

[9] Mebs D. Venomous and poisonous animals. Stuttgart (Germany): Medpharm Scientific Publishers; 2002.

[10] Dart RC, McNally J. Efficacy, safety and use of snake antivenoms in the United States. Ann Emerg Med 2001;37(2):181–8.

[11] Clark RF. The safety and efficacy of antivenin *Latrodectus mactans*. J Toxicol Clin Toxicol 2001;39:125–7.

[12] Gibly R, Williams M, Walter FG, et al. Continuous intravenous midazolam infusion for *Centruroides exilicauda* scorpion envenomation. Ann Emerg Med 1999;34:620–5.

[13] Seifert SA, et al. Position statement: institutions housing venomous animals. J Med Toxicol 2006;2(3):118–9.

ELSEVIER
SAUNDERS

VETERINARY
CLINICS
Exotic Animal Practice

Vet Clin Exot Anim 11 (2008) 403–421

Index

Note: Page numbers of article titles are in **boldface** type.

A

ABCs, of emergency management of toxicoses, 212–217
    airway interventions in, 212, 214–215
    assisted ventilation in, 213–215
    blood pressure assessment in, 213, 219
    breathing interventions in, 212, 214–215
    cardiopulmonary-cerebral resuscitation in, 213–215
    circulation in, 213–217
    hypovolemic hypotension treatment in, 214–217
    perfusion assessment in, 213
    pulse assessment in, 213, 216
    supplemental oxygen treatment in, 212–213, 215

Abdominal radiographs, for zinc toxicosis, 222–223
    in domestic rabbit toxicoses, 318–319

Acetaminophen toxicity, emergency management of, 226
    in ferrets, 310

N-Acetylcysteine (Mucomyst), for ferret toxicology, 310

Acid reducers, for ferret toxicology, 307–308

Acidic toxins, corrosive, in ferret toxicology, 302–303
    cleaning products as, 304–305

Activated charcoal, for aquarium fish toxicology, 367
    for domestic rabbit toxicoses, 317
    for ferret toxicology, 302–304, 307, 311
    for heavy metal exposures, 223
    for insecticide exposures, 225
    for oral exposure decontamination, 220
    for pet bird toxicity, 239, 241, 250
    for raptor toxicology, 272

Aeration, water, for aquarium fish toxicology, 364–365, 369

Aerosols, in pet bird toxicity, 233
    pesticide, in aquarium fish toxicology, 369

Aflatoxins, in aquarium fish toxicology, 371
    in domestic rabbit toxicoses, 323
    in pet bird toxicity, 245–246
    in waterfowl toxicology, 294

Agitation, emergency management of, 218

Air fresheners, in pet bird toxicity, 233

Airborne toxins. See also *Inhaled toxins.*
    in pet bird toxicity, 230–233
        miscellaneous, 233
        nicotine as, 232–233
        polytetrafluoroethylene as, 230–231
        smoke as, 231–232

Airway interventions, in emergency management of toxicoses, 212, 214–215

Alcohol-based products, in ferret toxicology, 307

Aldrin, in waterfowl toxicology, 292

Algae, blooms of, in waterfowl toxicology, 295
    water quality–related, in aquarium fish toxicology, 364, 373

Algicides, in aquarium fish toxicology, 373

Alkaline toxins, corrosive, in ferret toxicology, 302–303
    cleaning products as, 304–305

Aluminum, diagnostic sampling for, 206
    in aquarium fish toxicology, 372

Amanitin, diagnostic sampling for, 202
    emergency management of toxicosis with, 222